BRITISH GERIATRIC MEDICINE
IN THE 1980s

British Geriatric Medicine
in the 1980s

KEITH ANDREWS AND JOHN BROCKLEHURST

King Edward's Hospital Fund for London

© King Edward's Hospital Fund for London 1987
Typeset by Tradespools Ltd, Frome, Somerset
Printed and bound in England by Hollen Street Press Ltd

ISBN 0 900 889 93 4

King's Fund Publishing Office
2 St Andrew's Place
London NW1 4LB

Preface

Geriatric medicine is now one of the major specialties within medicine in Great Britain and Northern Ireland. This development has come about in just over 35 years and marks a response to striking demographic changes. While other developed societies have had to meet similar demographic changes, they have generally been slower in developing geriatrics as a specialty and in some cases have been opposed to such a development. British leadership in this field has sprung from three main causes: the historical legacy of major state participation in care of the elderly since the Poor Relief Act of 1601; a striking absence (until the last few years) of a private sector in this field; and above all the inception in 1948 of the National Health Service.

Since there is no simple or generally accepted definition of a geriatric patient, services might be expected to vary considerably in different parts of the country. For administrative simplicity in regard to emergency admission of old people to hospital, general physicians and geriatricians have in many cases agreed to an age cut-off for emergency admissions to either general medicine or geriatrics. This varies from 65 to 80 years. However, many old people admitted to hospital are not acute emergencies but patients in whom breakdown in independent living has been occurring over days, weeks or even months. These will become geriatric patients not because of an age limit but because of the complex nature of this breakdown, often involving a background of ageing, multiple pathology and social deprivation and a precipitating event, either medical or social. The specialty of geriatric medicine may therefore be seen more in terms of the organisation of a system of medical care rather than on an age-defined basis. It provides facilities for medical diagnosis and treatment, rehabilitation, community support through day hospital and other means, and also long-term care.

Because of this complexity of presentation and the variation in provisions and patterns which inevitably follow, and also because geriatrics has been acknowledged by successive governments as a priority area within health care, it seems timely to survey the resources available to the specialty and the different ways in which these are deployed.

The present volume is based on a series of four different questionnaires as well as personal visits to 36 departments throughout the country. It gives an overview of geriatrics today from which we have drawn out what we believe are important issues for future development.

We gratefully acknowledge the excellent cooperation which we have had from our colleagues in geriatrics, nursing, physiotherapy and occupational therapy in undertaking this work. Without their ready response the information on which the studies are based would not have materialized. We would wish to acknowledge also the helpful information we have received from Mrs Audrey Miller relating to her study of primary nursing in geriatrics. We are grateful to Ms Kathleen Harrison who has borne the brunt of the manuscript preparation and to the King's Fund for financial assistance in carrying out these studies.

Keith Andrews
John Brocklehurst
Manchester
1987

Note

Some of the material presented here has been reported in a much briefer form in the scientific literature. This volume develops the themes and expands on certain data previously reported in the following publications.

British Medical Journal (1984) Provision of remedial therapists in geriatric medicine. 289:661.
Age and Ageing (1985) Geriatric medicine—the style of practice. 14:1–7.
Journal of the Royal College of Physicians of London (1985) The implications of demographic changes on resource allocation. 19:109–111.
Journal of the Royal College of Physicians of London (1985) A profile of geriatric rehabilitation units. 19:240–242.
International Rehabilitation Medicine (1985) What would physiotherapists do if they had more staff? 6:785–786.
International Rehabilitation Medicine (1985) What would occupational therapists do if they had more staff? 7:137–139.
Nursing Times (1987) Nurse staffing in geriatric wards. Occasional paper 83:48–51.

Contents

1	Organisation	13
2	Resources	19
3	Rehabilitation	35
4	Long-term care	44
5	Variations in the style of geriatric practice	53
6	Nurse provision	61
7	Occupational therapy	73
8	Physiotherapy	86
9	Conclusions	103
	References	114
	Index	117

TABLES

1	Relationship of age with hospital admission and length of stay	20
2	Regional bed provision in geriatric medicine	21
3	Discharge rate related to number of beds per population	22
4	Geriatric practice throughout the UK	22
5	Discharges related to proportion of long-stay beds in the geriatric unit	23
6	Regional consultant manpower and beds in geriatric medicine	24
7	Beds per consultant geriatrician in the UK	24
8	Discharges from geriatric units related to number of consultants per population	25
9	Discharges related to number of beds per consultant geriatrician	25
10	Relationship of number of consultant geriatricians per unit to available resources	26
11	Therapy staff in geriatric departments	28
12	Discharges from geriatric units in the UK	28
13	Discharges related to bed provision in geriatric units	29

14	Discharges per bed related to beds per population	29
15	Sources of admission of patients admitted to rehabilitation wards	36
16	Age and sex distribution of admissions to rehabilitation units	37
17	Implications of demographic changes for annual bed-days occupied on rehabilitation wards in 36 units	37
18	Diagnoses of admissions and discharges on rehabilitation wards	39
19	Length of stay of patients discharged from rehabilitation wards	40
20	Placement of discharged rehabilitation patients	40
21	Follow-up arrangements for patients discharged from rehabilitation wards	41
22	Teaching on rehabilitation wards	42
23	Admissions to long-stay wards	45
24	Median length of stay on long-stay wards by age and sex	46
25	Median length of stay on long-stay wards by main diagnosis	46
26	Day-to-day responsibility on long-stay wards	47
27	Time spent per week by medical staff in long-stay wards	48
28	Frequency of consultant ward rounds in long-stay wards	49
29	Activities and resources for long-stay patients with and without separate accommodation	49
30	Styles of geriatric units in the UK	54
31	Sources of admission to different types of ward a) admissions from the community	54
32	Sources of admission to different types of ward b) intra-hospital transfers	55
33	Length of stay in different types of geriatric wards	56
34	Type of service compared with resources and discharge rate	56
35	Resources in different types of geriatric units	57
36	Staff levels in different types of geriatric units	58
37	Numbers of departments and types of service in different population groups	58
38	Special organisations associated with geriatric units	59
39	Beds per nurse at different times of the day	62
40	Occupied beds per nurse in different types of wards at various times throughout a 24-hour period	65

Contents

41	Number of occupied beds and nurses on duty in different types of wards at 9.30am	65
42	Comparison of trained and untrained nurses and learners in different types of wards	66
43	Trained nursing staff on duty at different times of the day	66
44	Dependency on nurses by geriatric patients	70
45	Occupational therapy staffing levels in geriatric units and therapists' opinions of adequacy of provision	75
46	Required occupational therapist levels according to staff satisfaction with present staffing levels	76
47	Occupational therapist staffing levels in geriatric medicine—present and required	76
48	Occupational therapists in geriatric medicine in the study area	77
49	Occupational therapists in geriatric units in the UK	78
50	Style of geriatric unit and occupational therapist staffing levels	79
51	Occupational therapist staffing levels related to geriatric unit characteristics	80
52	Proportion of time spent on different activities by trained occupational therapists	81
53	Discharge planning	82
54	Proportion of treatment time spent on different activities by trained occupational therapists	82
55	Areas of increased activity if more occupational therapists were available	84
56	Provision of aids	85
57	Physiotherapy staffing on geriatric units related to therapists' opinions of adequacy of staffing levels	88
58	Physiotherapist levels according to staff satisfaction with present staffing levels	88
59	Physiotherapist staffing levels in geriatric medicine—present and required	89
60	Physiotherapists in geriatric medicine in the study area	89
61	Physiotherapy staff in geriatric units throughout the UK	90
62	Style of geriatric unit and physiotherapist staffing levels	91
63	Physiotherapy staffing levels related to geriatric unit characteristics	92

64	Proportion of time spent on different activities by trained physiotherapists	93
65	Areas of increased activity if more physiotherapists were available	94
66	Physiotherapy equipment used in geriatric units	96
67	Frequency of use of walking aids in geriatric rehabilitation	97
68	Equipment used in treating pressure sores	97
69	Rehabilitation techniques used in stroke therapy	98
70	Equipment used in stroke rehabilitation	99
71	Slings used for arm support in hemiplegia	100
72	Distances between geriatric units and limb-fitting centres	100
73	Assessment for wheelchair provision	100

FIGURES

1	Scattergram of consultants per population by region	23
2	Scattergram of physiotherapists and occupational therapists per population by region	27
3	Sample recreation unit activities programme	50
4	Ratio of beds per nurse	63
5	Beds per nurse, beds per trained nurse and percentage of beds occupied in different types of wards	64
6	Beds per nurse, beds per trained nurse and percentage of beds occupied in different types of geographical areas	67

1 Organisation

Introduction

Geriatric medicine specialises in the management of disease and disability occurring in elderly people. The main difference from general medicine is its organisational approach to the provision of services. Whereas general medicine is able to provide management of medical conditions in either an acute medical ward or an outpatient clinic, geriatric medicine has an armamentarium of acute, rehabilitation and long-stay facilities, day hospitals, intermittent or relief admissions, domiciliary physiotherapy and a close liaison with the community and social service departments.

There has been a swift expansion of geriatric medicine over the last 35 years. This rapid development has inevitably resulted in a variety of approaches to the organisation of the specialty. Each area has developed its own style of practice depending on a number of factors such as the distribution of beds, local resources, the needs and pressures of the community being served and the particular interests and training of the geriatrician in charge. As the studies described in this book show, there is wide variation between health districts as well as between the four countries which make up the UK. This is particularly apparent in the provision of geriatric beds, influenced largely by the provision of long-stay residential care. Those requiring medical and nursing supervision are generally regarded as being the responsibility of the hospital services (funded nationally) whereas those requiring social supervision are the responsibility of the social service departments (funded locally). There is, however, no clear line of distinction between these two types of provision and each district has a different threshold for the acceptance of the various forms of care. In Scotland there is a lower provision of social service residential care than in England and Wales, but the geriatric bed provision is higher. In Northern Ireland the geriatric beds and social service provision are basically the responsibility of the same authority and therefore they appear to have a higher number of geriatric beds with a larger number of long-stay patients than England and Wales.

The social service residential homes are coming under increasing pressure to accept more heavily dependent individuals[1]. In general they have neither the staff nor the expertise to cope with many of the problems of the elderly. The staff are naturally unhappy to transfer to a long-stay hospital ward an elderly person for whom they have been caring when there is a deterioration in the physical or mental state. This attachment to the elderly person and the recognition that the residential home is indeed the patient's home is commendable but does result in difficulty in providing appropriate levels of care, with misplacement in both residential homes and in hospital[2]. A few homes jointly funded by health and social services departments have developed a greater level of nursing care as a solution. They need careful monitoring, however, to ensure that they do not become inadequately provided mini-hospitals.

The planning of services has been further complicated by the rapid expansion of private rest and nursing homes. Private rest homes are the equivalent of the social service residential homes providing social care with no requirement to have nursing staff on duty. Private nursing homes must have nurses on duty and can accept more heavily dependent patients requiring nursing and medical care. There has been some concern that these homes do not necessarily provide support for the same client groups as the health and social service departments. This is particularly relevant, since health authorities take the presence of private homes into account when assessing local bed provision for geriatric services. There is also concern about the problems that would be created for the hospital and social service departments should a private institution have to close suddenly. In addition there has been a great deal of publicity about neglect in some homes and the lack of control over the quality of care provided.

Another element in the planning of services is the amount of community support available. The present trend is to move the emphasis from hospital care to management in the community. This is taking place at a time when the provision of residential places[3], meals-on-wheels[4] and home help services[5] is progressively falling behind the demographic trends. Unless there is an appropriate increase in the provision of community services to enable a satisfactory transfer of care to the community, more problems will be created than solved.

The development of resources in geriatric units is thus taking place against a varied background of other forms of provision for the elderly. Each district will therefore develop a different type of service.

Historical background

Geriatric medicine began its life as an organised and recognised specialty with the inception of the National Health Service in 1948. During the previous 10 to 15 years a handful of pioneers had been exploring ways of improving the lot of those patients suffering from the effects of ageing and chronic disease who were eking out the last years of their lives in chronic sick wards of general hospitals and in workhouse infirmaries. The acknowledged pioneer is Dr Marjorie Warren, who worked at the West Middlesex Hospital and its associated workhouse infirmary. With the inception of the NHS it became possible for specialists to be appointed as consultant geriatricians and these appointments have gradually continued until virtually every health district in Great Britain now has a geriatric service headed by one or more consultants. At the latest count there are about 500 consultant geriatricians in Great Britain.

The first generation of consultant geriatricians when appointed were made responsible for between 200 and 400 beds, usually spread over three, four or five different hospitals, all completely full and with the addition of a waiting list, very often of similar size to the number of beds. Many of the patients in these beds had been transferred from the acute wards of general hospitals and from the teaching hospitals (at that time an élite); others had been admitted direct from the workhouse with acute episodes of disease. In many cases, little attempt had been made at rehabilitation or restoration of function before the patients were committed to chronic sick wards and workhouse infirmaries and there was virtually no ongoing medical input or physical therapy in the wards and infirmaries themselves. The newly appointed consultant's first task, therefore, would be to examine all the patients in the beds under his care to decide which had remediable problems, and to restore them to independence wherever possible. This involved both a careful medical examination and the implementation of some form of rehabilitation.

The second task facing the newly appointed consultant would be to become acquainted with those who were on the waiting list (many of whom may have been on it for over a year). He would visit all of these patients in their own homes or in hospitals where they might be waiting, in order to determine whether alternatives might be considered or to decide priority as far as transfer to geriatric beds was concerned. On reviewing the waiting list in this way it would be apparent that many individuals had died or moved elsewhere and that for others some form of acute intervention might prevent the need for long-term care. The consultant would then admit, to those beds which became free, the patients whom he regarded as most likely to be restored to independent living through rehabilitation, following a careful medical, functional and social assessment. The later development of day hospitals allowed many patients to be rehabilitated, either without hospital admission at all or by an earlier discharge than might otherwise have been possible. In this way were established the main elements of geriatric care—domiciliary assessment, acute assessment, rehabilitation, the day hospital and long-term care. By these means, over the 38 years between 1948 and 1986 the numbers of geriatric beds have gradually diminished, waiting lists have disappeared, and long-term care, while remaining an important element in geriatric medicine, is no longer the dominant part.

As these various developments occurred, different hospitals would present themselves as especially appropriate to certain types of care. For instance, wards situated within a general hospital with easy access to diagnostic facilities would clearly be the most appropriate place for the acute admission and assessment of patients at the time of referral. Wards in a hospital where there was a strong occupational therapy and physiotherapy service would appear to be the most appropriate for rehabilitation. Small hospitals and others scattered over a wider area would lend themselves particularly to long-term care for individuals who could then be closer to their own communities. Each consultant would organise his service according to the resources that were available to him and to local need. Pressures on him would include not only the beds and day hospital facilities in his own charge, but also their numbers in relation to general medical beds, places in residential (Part III) homes, any private care that was available, and the contribution made by the psychiatric service to the management of old people. The latter has developed particularly over the last 10 to 15 years with the emergence of psychogeriatrics as an independent specialty. The creation of a small number of units for younger disabled people created the need for geriatricians to look after younger disabled patients.

The present investigation

Since these developments occurred over a wide front and offered many variations, and since resources have by no means been equally distributed throughout the country, it seemed important to take stock of the organisation and resources in geriatric departments in the 1980s. This book is, therefore, an account of the findings of a number of studies undertaken through 1982–83 which have been supported financially by the King's Fund. The studies involved a series of four postal questionnaires, followed by personal visits made by the authors to 36 different geriatric departments throughout the country.

Organisation

In the first study, questionnaires were sent to all consultant geriatricians and replies sought from each of the 272 geriatric departments. Two hundred and twelve replied—a 77 per cent response rate. This provided information on the number of consultants in the department; the population aged 65 and over who were served; the total number of beds and the distribution of these beds among acute, rehabilitation and long-stay care wards; the total deaths and discharges in 1981; further details about rehabilitation including the number of therapists in post, the provision of any special units (for example orthogeriatric or stroke rehabilitation units); the doctor in day-to-day charge of the patients; and the availability of any other special resources, such as psychogeriatrics and domiciliary physiotherapy.

In the second study, questionnaires completed by 54 departments involved a detailed appraisal of patients admitted to and discharged from geriatric rehabilitation and long-stay wards during a specific two-week period in 1983. These were only sent to departments which had specially designated rehabilitation or long-stay wards and which indicated from the first questionnaire a willingness to take part in this more detailed study. This second questionnaire provided the numbers of patients transferred to rehabilitation wards, together with the type of ward or place from which they had originated; the main diagnosis; and the age and sex. For those discharged from the rehabilitation wards, respondents indicated the total length of inpatient stay, where they were discharged to and what follow-up arrangements had been made. It also involved a similar statement about patients transferred to long-term care beds, including the type of ward from which they had come (or whether it was their own home or other community facility) and the length of stay in the geriatric unit up to the time of admission to the long-term care bed. Similarly, information was obtained about those patients discharged from long-stay wards. In addition the total number of hours of medical input into rehabilitation and long-stay wards of staff of all grades in the two-week period was recorded.

In the third and fourth studies, questionnaires were sent to the senior physiotherapists and occupational therapists in all the geriatric departments in the UK. Replies were received from 196 (73 per cent) of the physiotherapy and 203 (76 per cent) of the occupational therapy departments. (There are 268 such departments within geriatric units. Units where therapy was provided from general hospital departments were excluded.) These provided information about the staff in post in all grades and also the therapists' view of the shortage of staff for requirements. It also provided information about the different types of equipment and the different management techniques used.

From these four studies it has been possible to build up a comprehensive picture of the state of geriatric medicine at the present time. To complete it, however, it was felt important to make personal visits to a representative series of departments throughout the country (the fifth study). Altogether, 36 different departments were visited by one or other of the authors. In each department a one in five sample of wards was visited (an average of five wards per department) and in each ward a one in two sample of the patients in the ward was taken to obtain information about age, length of stay and principal diagnosis. On these visits, the number of nurses on duty at different times on the day of the visit was also recorded. This information helped to demonstrate how closely the patients in the different types of geriatric wards conformed to the description of the ward (acute, rehabilitation, long-stay or mixed) and also provided a profile of nurse staffing in different types of geriatric wards based on the numbers of nurses working in the wards.

All these findings have been brought together in the present volume and the main conclusions and recommendations are summarised in the last chapter. It is hoped that these findings will provide a factual basis for forward planning as well as comprising a view of the organisation and resources of British geriatric medicine in the 1980s.

2 Resources

Introduction

At the inception of the NHS in 1948 there were only five or six physicians in Great Britain involved in services specially designed for the needs of the elderly. By 1983, over 500 consultant physicians were practising completely, or predominantly, in geriatric medicine. This growth rate is remarkable, particularly when compared with other countries where geriatric medicine is still a new medical specialty.

Geriatric medicine is principally an organisational specialty within general medicine. The consultant is responsible for the organisation and management of a system of care whose primary aim is to accept old people at the point at which their independence is threatened and, through processes of assessment, rehabilitation and continuing support (including day care), to restore them and maintain them in the community. If this primary objective fails, the geriatric service then provides the great majority of long-term hospital care for the elderly.

In the years since the inception of the NHS, organisational variations have developed according to local needs and resources. Varying styles of practice have developed in relation to acute, rehabilitation and long-stay beds (see chapter 5). Each department of course has an obligation to deploy its resources to provide an optimal service for the population it serves.

This chapter considers the overall pattern of resource provision in the geriatric service in Great Britain, noting regional and other variations, how staff in post match the recommended figures of various reports and to what extent variation in staffing and practice is reflected in patient turnover.

The findings reported here are principally derived from the first study (see chapter 1). The questionnaire used provided for the following information:
   population aged 65-plus served by the unit
   total number of beds
   total deaths and discharges in 1981
   staff in post at the time the questionnaire was completed (doctors, physiotherapists, occupational therapists, and social workers).
Altogether, consultants from 212 departments of geriatric medicine

completed the questionnaire—a response rate of 77 per cent (varying from 56 per cent in the South East Thames region to 92 per cent in Trent region). The population aged 65 and over served by the 212 departments numbers 6.5 million (a figure which conforms well with the total UK population aged 65 and over of 8.3 million). In the very small number of cases where a department consists of consultants practising in general and geriatric medicine, the figures relate only to the geriatric beds.

Patients

Information about individual patients was obtained for a sample of 2,151 patients in 36 different units in study 5. The percentage of these patients in different age groups is shown in Table 1. This

Table 1 Relationship of age with hospital admission and length of stay

	Type of ward*												
	A		R		L		A/R		R/L		A/R/L		Total	
	$x†$	$y‡$	x	y	x	y	x	y	x	y	x	y	x	y
Male (n = 665)														
<65	2	1	2	11	5	9	0	0	1	3	2	<1	3	7
−74	23	18	26	20	35	38	47	61	30	21	27	18	30	32
−84	59	61	49	47	43	38	35	21	45	52	53	59	48	44
⩾85	16	19	23	22	17	14	18	18	23	24	18	21	19	17
Female (n = 1486)														
<65	1	1	1	1	1	2	2	1	0	0	<1	<1	1	2
−74	13	24	20	34	12	11	17	19	10	10	15	9	14	12
−84	62	59	48	39	47	44	48	58	59	45	58	65	52	47
⩾85	24	16	30	26	40	43	32	22	30	45	26	26	32	40
Total (n = 2151)														
<65	1	1	2	4	2	4	1	1	<1	1	1	<1	2	3
−74	16	22	22	30	18	17	24	26	19	13	20	12	19	17
−84	61	60	48	41	46	43	45	52	53	47	56	63	51	46
⩾85	22	17	28	25	34	36	29	21	27	40	23	24	28	34

The table shows the percentage of patients in various age groups on different types of ward and the percentage of hospital days occupied by each age group on each ward.
† x = per cent of ward population
‡ y = per cent of hospital days occupied

*NB Throughout this book the following abbreviations are used to indicate different types of wards: A—acute; R—rehabilitation; L—long-stay. Combinations are represented as follows: AR/L—combined acute and rehabilitation with separate long-stay; A/R/L—separate acute, rehabilitation and long-stay; ARL—combined acute, rehabilitation and long-stay; AR/L—combined acute and rehabilitation with separate long-stay; RL—combined rehabilitation and long-stay only.

indicates that altogether 79 per cent of patients in geriatric wards were aged 75 and over (28 per cent were aged 85 and over). There is some variation in relation to different types of wards but this is minimal and is as follows:

Acute and rehabilitation combined 74 per cent
Rehabilitation only 76 per cent
Acute, rehabilitation and long-term care
combined 79 per cent
Long-stay only or combined with rehabilitation 80 per cent
Acute only 83 per cent

It is notable that the acute wards have the highest proportion of patients aged 75 and over. Table 1 also shows the percentage of hospital days occupied by the different age groups. Eighty per cent are in patients aged 75 and over and 34 per cent in patients aged 85 and over.

Beds

Table 2 shows the proportion of geriatric beds per 1000 population aged 65 and over; it varies from 6.10 in South West Thames to 13.12 in Scotland. The mean figure for the UK is 8.30. Altogether 34 per

Table 2   Regional bed provision in geriatric medicine (1982)

Region	Departments contacted	Replies (%)	Total population	Beds/ population	% with <7.5 beds/ population
North West	22	91	595.1	8.21	35
Mersey	12	67	218.8	8.34	25
West Midlands	21	71	462.8	9.58	27
Trent	13	92	585.3	7.56	23
Yorkshire	20	75	460.0	8.89	27
Northern	19	79	371.2	7.70	40
Oxford	8	88	269.6	7.32	57
South West	14	71	353.6	7.09	50
Wessex	7	71	239.6	7.73	60
East Anglia	10	90	356.3	7.50	44
SW Thames	15	87	424.1	6.10	70
SE Thames	18	56	357.7	6.98	30
NE Thames	21	76	433.1	7.98	44
NW Thames	15	73	317.4	6.32	73
England	215	76	5444.6	7.59	41
Wales	18	72	321.5	9.10	8
Scotland	30	87	639.9	13.12	4
N Ireland	11	73	137.6	12.27	13
Total	274	77	6543.6	8.30	34

cent of the departments had fewer than 7.5 beds per population* and 5 per cent less than 4.5 beds; 7 per cent had more than 13.5 beds per population.

The optimal discharge rate occurs in those areas with 7.6 to 10.5 beds per population (Table 3) and the discharge rate diminishes

---

*NB Throughout this book population is defined as 1000 persons aged 65 and over.

Table 3 Discharge rate related to number of beds per population

Beds/population	Number of departments	Discharge/population Mean	SD
<4.5	8	15.4	5.9
4.5–6	18	26.2	11.7
6.1–7.5	34	26.2	18.4
7.6–9	56	45.7	17.6
9.1–10.5	29	41.6	17.5
10.6–12	11	34.7	13.7
12.1–13.5	15	23.9	10.2
>13.5	11	23.9	10.2
Insufficient data	30		

both when there are fewer beds and when there are more. The various bed provisions throughout the UK led to a development of different methods of practice and this can be seen to some extent when looking at the proportion of beds that are used for long-stay care (Table 4). The mean figure for the UK is 55 per cent of geriatric beds for long-term care—but there is great variation between the different countries (50 per cent in England to 74–75 per cent in Scotland and Northern Ireland). These national differences indicate fundamental differences in policy regarding geriatric beds—both

Table 4 Geriatric practice throughout the UK

	England	Wales	Scotland	N. Ireland	UK
Beds/population					
No of units	160	13	26	8	207
Mean beds/population	7.74	9.68	13.28	11.80	8.71
SEM	0.16	0.51	0.61	1.18	0.41
<6	19%	0	4%	0	15%
–7.5	25%	8%	0	13%	20%
–9	34%	38%	0	0	29%
–10.5	15%	23%	12%	13%	15%
–13.5	8%	30%	35%	63%	15%
>13.5	0	0	50%	13%	7%
% Beds which are long-stay					
No of units	133	12	25	8	178
Mean % beds for long-stay	49.9	58.8	73.8	75.4	55.0
S.E.M.	1.5	6.4	1.8	1.8	1.4
<40%	27%	25%	0	0	22%
–60%	43%	25%	12%	0	35%
>60%	30%	50%	88%	100%	43%

Scotland and Northern Ireland include in their complement what in England would be residential home (Part III) beds. As might be expected, the greater the proportion of long-stay beds the lower the discharge rate (Table 5).

Resources

Table 5 Discharges related to the proportion of long-stay beds in the geriatric unit

	Number of units	Mean discharges/ population	SEM
% Beds long-stay			
<40	32	44.2	5.7
−60	58	42.4	5.3
>60	68	29.6	1.8

Consultants

The mean number of consultant geriatricians per 1000 population aged 65 plus varies from .039 in East Anglia to .095 in Northern Ireland (Table 6). The overall mean figure for the UK is .066. The proportion of departments with fewer than .07 consultants per 1000 population aged 65 plus varies from 100 per cent in the South West to 25 per cent in Northern Ireland. The distribution of consultants by region is shown in a scattergram in Figure 1.

Figure 1 Scattergram of consultants per population by region

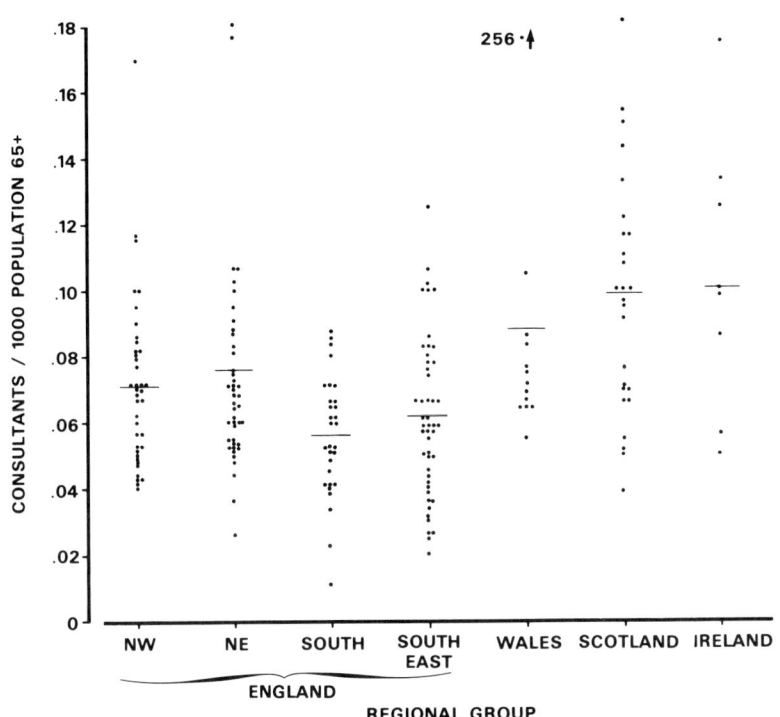

Table 6 also shows the number of beds per consultant, which varies from 105 in the Mersey region to 152 in Wessex. The overall average is 131. The proportion of departments with more than 140 beds per consultant varies from 60 per cent in Wessex to 13 per cent

Table 6 Regional consultant manpower and beds in geriatric medicine (1982)

		Departments replying		
	Consultants/ population	% with <.07 consultants/ population	Beds/ consultant	% departments with >140 beds/consultant
Region				
North West	.074	55	115	30
Mersey	.087	33	105	13
West Midlands	.065	60	146	40
Trent	.058	85	136	38
Yorkshire	.062	47	149	47
Northern	.084	33	106	13
Oxford	.059	57	119	29
South West	.051	100	142	60
Wessex	.050	80	152	60
East Anglia	.039	56	121	23
SW Thames	.052	54	111	23
SE Thames	.050	80	149	40
NE Thames	.062	67	125	25
NW Thames	.054	82	128	27
England	.062	61	128	23
Wales	.078	46	125	38
Scotland	.092	27	151	50
N Ireland	.095	25	145	38
Total	.066	55	131	35

in Mersey and Northern regions. About one quarter of consultants were looking after more than 160 beds (Table 7). That the number of consultants per population affects the discharge rate is shown in Table 8 where optimum discharge rates are obtained with a rate of .071 to .089 (equivalent to one consultant per 1123 to 1400

Table 7 Beds per consultant geriatrician in the UK

	England	Wales	Scotland	N Ireland	UK
No of units	165	13	26	8	212
Mean beds/ consultant	128.0	125.3	151.4	145.1	131.3
SEM	4.9	10.2	12.2	37.8	4.4
<100	28%	31%	31%	50%	30%
−160	48%	46%	31%	25%	45%
>160	24%	23%	38%	25%	25%

population aged 65 and over). Relating discharges to the number of beds per geriatrician (Table 9) again shows an optimal rate at 101–140 and less. The fall-off at high levels is presumably due to the greater scope for accommodating long-stay patients (see above).

The number of consultants per department might be expected to vary with the nature of the department, its catchment area and its responsibilities for undergraduate teaching. The range is from one to seven consultants. The figures (from 214 respondents) are as follows:

one consultant	65 (30.4 per cent)
two consultants	99 (46.3 per cent)
three consultants	30 (14.0 per cent)
four or more consultants	20 (8.5 per cent)

Table 10 shows, as might be expected, that the more consultants per department, the better the resources (fewer population and beds per consultant and more beds per population). There is also an increase in some performance indicators, such as the number of discharges per bed per year and discharges per 1000 population aged 65 plus per year (Table 10).

Table 8 Discharges from geriatric units related to the number of consultants per population (186 departments)

Consultants/ population	Number of departments	Discharges/population Mean	SD
<0.04	15	24.8	11.5
−0.05	17	33.3	9.8
−0.06	39	36.3	18.5
−0.07	34	40.0	17.3
−0.08	25	43.1	20.4
−0.09	15	40.7	28.8
−0.11	18	40.7	15.9
>0.11	21	39.1	22.8

Table 9 Discharges related to the number of beds per consultant geriatrician

Beds/consultant	Number of units	Mean	SEM
<100	50	39.8	3.4
−140	63	42.0	2.1
−180	45	36.0	2.5
>180	27	28.2	2.7

Table 10 Relationship of number of consultant geriatricians per unit to available resources

No of consultants per unit	1	2	3	≥4
Consultants/population				
n	63	95	30	20
Mean (SD)	0.063 (.036)	0.074 (.030)	0.082 (.033)	0.097 (.033)
<.07 consultants/population	78%	55%	40%	20%
Beds/consultant				
Mean (SD)	153.6 (61.0)	125.2 (44.8)	121.2 (40.0)	103.8 (40.8)
>140 beds/consultant	52%	30%	30%	15%
Beds/population				
Mean (SD)	8.7 (3.4)	8.5 (2.8)	9.0 (2.3)	9.4 (3.0)
<7.5 beds/population	35%	40%	23%	25%
Physiotherapists (PT)/population				
Mean (SD)	0.14 (0.09)	0.14 (0.08)	0.16 (0.15)	0.17 (0.11)
<0.15 PT/pop	70%	60%	55%	59%
Occupational therapists (OT)/population				
Mean (SD)	0.10 (0.06)	0.10 (0.07)	0.10 (0.09)	0.12 (0.07)
with no OT	7%	2%	0	0
<0.05 OT/pop	23%	21%	34%	6%
Social workers/population				
Mean (SD)	0.09 (0.06)	0.09 (0.05)	0.07 (0.05)	0.10 (0.08)
Discharges/bed/year				
Mean (SD)	4.2 (2.3)	4.7 (2.2)	4.9 (2.5)	5.4 (3.7)
>7.5 discharges/bed	7%	11%	14%	20%
Discharges/population				
Mean (SD)	34.7 (21.0)	38.1 (17.6)	41.5 (17.9)	41.5 (21.8)
<discharges/pop	30%	17%	10%	7%

Therapists

Resources available to geriatric departments in terms of physiotherapists and occupational therapists are shown in Tables 10 and 11. 'Total' therapists includes both trained therapists and untrained aides. The distribution of therapists by region is shown in a scattergram in Figure 2.

The average for trained physiotherapists is 0.14 per 1000 population aged 65 plus, varying from 0.082 in East Anglia to 0.19 in South Western. For total physiotherapy staff the mean is 0.24 per 1000 population aged 65 plus and the variations from 0.13 in East Anglia to 0.37 in Northern Ireland.

For trained occupational therapists the average is 0.10, varying from 0.07 per 1000 population aged 65 plus in North Western to 0.16 in SW Thames. For total occupational therapy staff the mean is 0.22 per 1000 population aged 65 plus, varying from 0.17 in the Northern region to 0.34 in Northern Ireland.

Figure 2 Scattergram of physiotherapists and occupational therapists per population by region

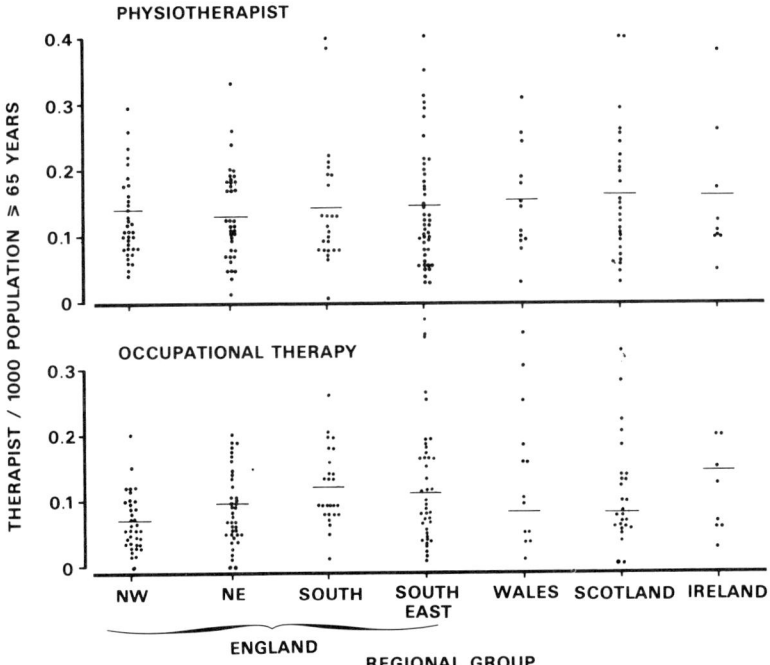

Comparing the provision of therapists to the number of consultants per department (Table 10) shows that the more consultants there are, the more there are trained physiotherapists per population. However such a relationship does not hold so directly for trained occupational therapists, or at all for social workers.

Table 11 shows regional variations in staff levels of therapists. The provision of therapists is dealt with in more detail in chapters 7 and 8.

Discharges

Table 12 shows the differences in discharge rate between the four countries. The units in Wales had the most rapid bed turnover, both

British Geriatric Medicine in the 1980s

Table 11 Therapy staff in geriatric departments (per population)

Region	Study population (000)	Physiotherapists Trained	Total	Occupational therapists Trained	Total
North Western	557.2	0.16	0.28	0.07	0.19
Mersey	176.8	0.12	0.19	0.09	0.19
West Midland	403.2	0.14	0.27	0.07	0.24
Trent	545.3	0.16	0.28	0.11	0.25
Yorkshire	460.0	0.13	0.27	0.08	0.22
Northern	312.2	0.10	0.18	0.06	0.17
Oxford	177.6	0.12	0.24	0.11	0.23
South Western	353.6	0.19	0.29	0.14	0.32
Wessex	176.0	0.10	0.15	0.12	0.19
East Anglia	356.3	0.08	0.13	0.09	0.19
SW Thames	359.1	0.18	0.23	0.16	0.22
SE Thames	367.7	0.11	0.20	0.07	0.19
NE Thames	411.1	0.11	0.21	0.10	0.22
NW Thames	280.7	0.14	0.21	0.12	0.26
England	4936.8	0.14	0.23	0.10	0.22
Wales	321.5	0.17	0.28	0.08	0.19
Scotland	639.9	0.17	0.23	0.11	0.20
N Ireland	137.6	0.17	0.37	0.15	0.34
Total	6035.8	0.14	0.24	0.10	0.22

Table 12 Discharges from geriatric units in the UK

	England	Wales	Scotland	N Ireland	UK
Discharges per population					
No of units	144	13	23	7	187
Mean discharges/population	38.8	56.7	26.4	21.2	37.8
SEM	1.4	8.3	3.2	3.6	1.4
<20	14%	0	43%	57%	19%
−40	43%	38%	39%	43%	43%
−60	28%	23%	18%	0	25%
>60	14%	38%	0	0	13%
Discharges per bed					
No of units	146	13	23	7	189
Mean discharges/bed	5.1	6.1	2.0	1.8	4.6
SEM	0.18	0.84	0.25	0.03	0.18
<4.5	47%	38%	96%	100%	55%
−9	47%	38%	4%	0	39%
>9	6%	23%	0	0	6%

in relation to population and to available beds. Scotland and Northern Ireland, with their higher number of beds per population, had lower discharge rates with very few departments achieving more than 4.5 discharges per bed and none more than 60 discharges per population. This confirms a greater deployment of geriatric beds on long-stay care in Scotland and Northern Ireland (see above).

Resources

When the discharges per population are correlated against beds per population (Table 13) the number of discharges rises as the number of beds increases up to 7.6–9 beds per population, after which there is a decrease in the discharge rate. The only figures which reach statistical significance are obtained when those units with less than 6 beds per population are compared with all the other groups up to 13.5 beds per population ($p<0.005$); and when those with more than 13.5 beds per population are compared with all the other groups above 6 beds per population ($p<0.05$).

Table 13   Discharges related to bed provision in geriatric units

		Discharges/population	
	Number of units	Mean	SEM
Beds/population			
<6	26	22.9	2.2
−7.5	34	38.3	3.2
−9	56	45.7	2.4
−10.5	29	41.6	3.2
−13.5	25	39.7	4.3
>13.5	11	23.9	3.3

When the discharges per bed are compared with the number of beds per population (Table 14) the number of discharges falls off after 9.01 beds per population. This difference is significant between the ranges of 9–10.5 and 6.01–7.5 beds per population ($p<0.05$), and between the ranges of 9.01–10.5 and 7.51–9 beds per population ($p<0.01$). The level of discharges per bed for the beds per population over 10.5 is significant against all the other ranges ($p<0.001$). Thus the number of discharges falls markedly for those units with more than 10.5 beds per 1000 population over the age of 65. One possible reason for this is that most of these units are in Scotland or Northern Ireland where the social service provision is either included in the geriatric bed provision (Northern Ireland) or there is a lower provision of social service homes (Scotland). In

Table 14   Discharges per bed related to beds per population

		Discharges/bed	
	Number of units	Mean	SEM
Beds/population			
<6	26	4.7	0.43
−7.5	34	5.6	0.53
−9	56	5.6	0.29
−10.5	29	4.3	0.33
>10.5	37	2.7	0.28

addition, these units tend to be in large geographical catchment areas which make community support more difficult to achieve and where the supportive value of the day hospital is more limited. There are, however, large variations within each group as can be seen by the standard deviations.

Discussion

That there should be considerable inequality in different districts in the numbers of consultants in post and the numbers of beds available is not surprising in a service which has developed rapidly and with only loosely applied central guidelines. While there are considerable mean differences between the regions in England, these are not great when compared with the difference between England and Wales on the one hand and Scotland and Northern Ireland on the other. The norm of geriatric beds proposed by the Department of Health and Social Security was, for many years, the round figure of 10 per 1000 people aged 65 and over, although the actual level of provision in 1980 was 8.1 per 1000 in England[1]. In 1983, however, the principle of national norms for resources in geriatric medicine was abandoned and it was left to health regions to make their own decisions. This they have done in their strategic plans and some of their figures are available. In a study of 14 draft ten-year regional strategic plans[2], 10 regions planned to provide between 6.0 and 8.5 beds per 1000 people aged 65 and over during the forthcoming decade.

In fact the number of beds available for geriatric medicine now is lower than it was in the 1950s and the whole development of the speciality has been set against a gradual saving in the number of beds[3]. In the face of a continuously growing population aged 65 plus, this indicates progressive efficiency in patient management. The average length of stay in departments of geriatric medicine fell by 4.5 per cent per year between 1972 and 1978 while the bed occupancy rate has remained steady at 92–93 per cent[1].

Our data show a mean of 8.3 beds per population with a wide variation between the different countries within the UK. England is lowest with 7.7 beds per population while Wales just about reaches the (previous) national norm at 9.7 beds per population. Scotland and Northern Ireland have higher starting norms, and although they do not reach these they have, on average, many more beds per population than either England or Wales. This can be seen particularly when the number of units with fewer than 7.5 beds per population is examined. In England as many as 44 per cent of units fell into this low figure compared with 4–13 per cent of the units in the other countries. Although the average figure for Northern Ireland was high there was a very wide variation in the range of beds per population—as many as 13 per cent of units had fewer than 7.5 beds per population while 13 per cent had over 13.5 beds per population.

The mean number of discharges per annum per 1000 population aged 65 plus is related to the number of beds per 1000 population aged 65 plus (Table 3). In England, with a small number of beds per population, only 30 per cent of units have more than 60 per cent of their beds used for long-term care compared with 50 per cent in Wales, 88 per cent in Scotland and all the units in Northern Ireland (Table 4). These levels are significant ($p<0.001$) when comparing units with under and over 60 per cent of all beds being used for long-stay care. The proportion of beds which are long-stay will obviously affect the discharge rate and this is confirmed by the marked drop in the discharges per population when more than 60 per cent of the beds are used for long-stay care (Table 5). This shows one of the variables in using length of stay or discharge rate as an evaluation of the effectiveness of geriatric units. Because it was not possible to obtain information about long-stay beds from those units without separate long-stay wards, this information refers to only 70 per cent of geriatric units.

The relevance of the different provisions of beds depends in part on local problems such as the availability of social service residential homes, private rest and nursing homes, family support and family attitudes, community support from district nurses, meals on wheels and home helps.

A problem in forecasting the number of beds required compared with population growth is the use of the age of 65 as the reference. The growth of the 65 plus age group has now plateaued and in general people aged 65 to 74 make little demand on the geriatric services—only 17 per cent of geriatric bed days (Table 1). Forward planning should therefore be based on the population aged 75 and over, who comprise 79 per cent of geriatric patients (Table 1); special weighting should also be given to those aged 85 and over, at present comprising 28 per cent of patients in geriatric wards (Table 1). In fact the proportion aged 75 plus will continue to rise throughout this century and the 85 plus age group will rise at an even faster rate. According to the registrar general's projections[4] the 75 plus group will grow by 28 per cent between 1981 and 2001 and the 85 plus group by 79 per cent. These age groups will contain those people in greatest need and most dependent on medical services.

Perhaps the most obvious performance indicator to use is the number of discharges per population per bed. This has considerable limitations in geriatric medicine. Variation in discharge rate may hide considerable differences in readmission rate. There is also variation in the extent to which geriatric beds are used for holiday relief admissions and other recurring short-term admissions. In addition, the responsibility of a geriatric service is not only to maintain a high discharge rate but to provide good quality long-term care and to ensure that aged people do not suffer by being discharged from hospital when they are not fit to live in the community. However, while accepting all these limitations discharge rate is probably the best measurement currently available to assess the efficiency of a geriatric service.

Based both on discharges per bed and discharges per population, the figure of 8.3 beds per population is the mean for optimal discharge rate in this study (that is, the mean of 7.6–9). This is the equivalent of 22 beds per 1000 population aged 75 and over and should be the minimal level to be aimed for. More beds probably allow greater flexibility in providing longer terms of treatment in hospital either for rehabilitation or long-stay care. The number of beds required will also depend on local community services and the availability of social service or private residential homes.

There are several norms quoted for the number of consultant geriatricians required for a given population. The British Medical Association working party[5] recommended levels of 0.107 consultants per 1000 population over the age of 65 while the British Geriatrics Society's[6] recommendations work out to the equivalent of 0.143 consultants per 1000 population over the age of 65. This study shows that figures for the UK in 1982–83 were very much less— 0.066 consultants per population. Even those regions with the highest ratio of consultants to the elderly population fall below these recommended levels. To reach the BMA norm, another 275 consultants would be needed to cover the 77 per cent of units which replied to this study (this figure includes 245 for England and Wales). Since these figures were collected there has been an increase in the number of consultants in geriatric medicine in England and Wales from 434 to 466 (in 1984), against a population aged 65 and over which numbered 7.5 million by 1984—a ratio of .062. It represents an average annual growth of 16 from 1979 to 1984. The BMA norm applied to the 1981 population aged 65 and over in England and Wales would require 803 consultants, compared with 466 in post in 1984. The higher figure is exactly the one quoted by the DHSS in 1981[7] as their target for the 1990s.

It is very difficult to decide what is a reasonable norm since there are so many influencing factors. We do not know how many of the consultants involved in the survey are practising in general as well as geriatric medicine. The proportion in England is small and is almost certainly reflected proportionately in our figures. In Scotland, Wales and Northern Ireland there are no such dual appointments. We suggest it is appropriate to regard consultants with dual appointments as contributing a full share to the geriatric services. They are involved only in multi-consultant units which are shown to score better on the performance indicators. Our data show that the discharge rate increases with the number of consultant geriatricians per population up to a level of about 0.08, after which the levels remain static (Table 8). Due to the small numbers involved and the wide variation within the groups these figures reach levels of statistical significance only for those areas where there are fewer than 0.04 consultants per population. Nevertheless there is a pattern which suggests that 0.08 consultants per population aged 65 plus are required. At present, 56 per cent of units in the UK fall below this level. More than 100 additional consultants would be required to bring all units up to the 0.08 standard. This would seem to be an immediate requirement before the higher norms are aimed for. The figure of 0.08 consultants per population aged 65 plus is equivalent to 0.21 consultants per population aged 75 plus.

Thirty per cent of geriatric departments have a single-handed geriatrician. These single-handed consultants are responsible for a larger total number of beds than their colleagues in multi-consultant units. They also have fewer beds per population and less physiotherapy per population (Table 9). There was no difference between the numbers of consultants per unit and the ratio of occupational therapists to the population, probably because all departments have very few occupational therapists. As many as 7 per cent of the single-handed geriatricians had no occupational therapist.

In view of these findings it is not surprising that in general the single-handed geriatricians have fewer discharges per bed and per 1000 population aged 65 plus, although there were large variations within each group. These figures suggest that the immediate concern must be to ensure that each district has at least two geriatricians.

Planning of geriatric hospital services should now be based on a unit of 1000 population aged 75 and over. The following norms are suggested as the most appropriate on the evidence presented here: 22 beds and 0.21 consultants (equivalent to 8.3 beds and 0.08 consultants per 1000 population aged 65 plus in 1981). This represents 67,500 beds and 650 consultants.

On these norms there was a shortfall of consultants in England and Wales of 137. On the basis of a growth rate of sixteen per annum (as during 1979 to 1984) the shortfall should be overcome within nine years. During that the time the population aged 75 and over may be expected to have risen by at least one million, indicating the need for a further 21 consultants. As far as beds are concerned, 79,000 would be required in England and Wales on 1981 census figures. The latest information available showed that there were 51,000 beds in England alone in 1982.

It is argued nowadays that no national norms are required and that each region should provide its own guidelines. It would seem essential if forward planning is to bear any rationality that resources for the elderly must be linked to population growth. Variables include the extent of provision of psycho-geriatric beds, private nursing home beds and places in residential homes (both statutory and private). These are likely to vary as much within regions as between regions and, while they must be taken into account, they would not seem to negate the need for some national guidelines.

3 Rehabilitation

Introduction

Rehabilitation is generally regarded as 'the restoration of the individual to his (or her) fullest physical, mental and social capability'[1] or 'the planned withdrawal of support'[2]. These definitions emphasise the important concepts of the multidisciplinary team approach, careful goal planning and continual assessment.

The pioneers of geriatric medicine recognised the importance of early mobilisation and for the patient to be actively involved in the normal routine of daily living. Thus patients were encouraged to get out of bed, to dress in day-time clothes and to take an interest in their appearance. This emphasis on functional recovery has become one of the hallmarks of good geriatric practice.

Rehabilitation in its broadest sense takes place throughout the whole process of geriatric care. Certain aspects of management, however, require the involvement of a multidisciplinary team and specific equipment, as opposed to medical and nursing 'care'.

Geriatricians have differing views as to the concept of rehabilitation in geriatric management. Some consider it to be the essential ingredient of any form of geriatric medicine and therefore regard it as illogical to have separate wards designated for rehabilitation. Others regard the educational philosophy of rehabilitation as being different from the medical-nursing model of management of the acutely ill patient or the social-nursing management of the long-stay patient. These geriatricians have designated specific wards for rehabilitation where the environment can be modified appropriately, where the nursing staff are orientated to the educational/rehabilitation style of management and specialised equipment is available.

As was shown in Chapter 2, about a quarter of geriatric units in our first study had separate wards designated for rehabilitation. In the second study further information was obtained from 36 of these units to demonstrate the characteristics of the wards and the workload they created.

During the two weeks of the study, 326 patients were discharged and 389 admitted to the rehabilitation wards of these 36 units. This was, on average, 6 to 7 patients admitted or discharged for each consultant—equivalent to 0.23 discharges and 0.28 admissions for each available rehabilitation bed.

Source of admission

About two thirds of admissions to the rehabilitation wards were direct from home (Table 15), 7 per cent of these from social service residential or private rest homes. It was rare for patients to be admitted directly from the accident and emergency department, probably because the primary assessment took place on the acute/assessment wards. This is supported by the finding that 13 per cent of admissions were from the acute/assessment geriatric wards.

Rehabilitation wards played an important role in the management of patients initially admitted to other hospital departments. About one fifth of patients on the rehabilitation wards had been transferred from other specialties, mainly medical (predominantly stroke patients) and orthopaedic (predominantly patients with fracture of the femur). However, apart from the orthopaedic units, few patients were transferred from surgical units.

Table 15 Sources of admission of patients admitted to rehabilitation wards

Source	Number of patients	%
From community		
Home	216	56
Social service home	22	6
Private rest home	5	1
Day hospital	4	1
Outpatient department	3	<1
Accident & emergency dept	3	<1
		65%
From hospital		
Acute geriatric unit	49	13
Long-stay ward	2	<1
Medical	31	8
Orthopaedic	38	10
Surgical	10	3
Psychiatry	1	<1
GP hospital	2	<1
Unknown	3	<1
		35%

The high proportion of patients transferred from orthopaedic units emphasises the importance of a close working relationship between the two specialties. Indeed, evidence from our first study suggests that about a quarter of geriatric units in the UK had a defined orthopaedic-geriatric liaison. In some cases this involved providing regular ward rounds on the orthopaedic wards. In a few units there was daily geriatric input to the orthopaedic wards, with early transfer of elderly orthopaedic patients to a specialised orthogeriatric unit where joint ward rounds by a geriatrician and an orthopaedic surgeon took place.

Age and sex distribution

It is generally thought by those not involved in geriatric medicine that the elderly are too frail to benefit from a physical programme. This view was obviously not held by geriatricians since the mean age of the patients on the rehabilitation wards was about 80 years for both males and females. Males accounted for 27 per cent of those admitted and 34 per cent of those discharged during the two-week study period (Table 16).

Table 16 Age and sex distribution of admissions to rehabilitation units

	Admissions			Discharges		
	Male	Female	Total	Male	Female	Total
Number	103	284	387	110	216	326
Age	%	%	%	%	%	%
<65	1	3	2	5	3	4
65–69	6	2	3	10	5	7
70–74	17	13	14	20	8	12
75–79	24	20	21	29	23	25
80–84	27	31	30	23	31	28
85–89	19	19	19	8	20	16
≥90	5	11	9	5	9	8
Not stated	2	1	1	0	0	0
Mean age	79.5	80.9	80.5	76.7	80.6	79.3
SEM	0.63	0.44	0.37	0.76	0.49	0.42

Primarily, the rehabilitation units were managing very old people. Although the ages ranged from below 65 to 99, 5 per cent of males and about 10 per cent of females were over 90, while four fifths of patients treated on the geriatric rehabilitation wards were over 75. This is important, since demographic changes suggest that the major population increases over the next 20 years will be in the 75 and over age groups.

The relevance of this is seen from our personal visits where we recorded the length of stay of a sample of patients on different types of wards in 36 units. The total bed-days occupied by these patients on the rehabilitation wards was 5260 for males and 18,394 for females (Table 17). Using the expected demographic trends for

Table 17 Implications of demographic changes for annual bed-days occupied on rehabilitation wards in 36 units

	Bed-days occupied in year			
	1981	1986	1996	2006
Males	5260	5593 (+6.3%) *	5935 (+12.8%)	5965 (+13.4%)
Females	18394	19366 (+5.3%)	20011 (+8.8%)	19490 (+6.0%)
All	23654	24959 (+5.5%)	25946 (+9.7%)	25455 (+7.6%)

*Figures in parentheses are % change from 1981.

males and females in different age bands[3], it has been possible to calculate the equivalent number of bed-days that will be occupied in these units over the next few decades (Table 17). The units studied can expect an additional 12.8 per cent bed-days for males and 8.8 per cent for females in 1996 than at the time of the study. This assumes that there is no change in the pattern of care. Of course there are a number of changes which might influence these figures up or down. Greater use of community support and domiciliary rehabilitation will decrease the need for more hospital places whereas a failure of the community services to keep pace with increasing need will result in a greater demand for hospital care and greater difficulty in discharging patients home.

Diagnosis

The most frequent diagnoses quoted for the patients admitted to and discharged from the rehabilitation wards in the second study are shown in Table 18. Multiple pathology is common in the elderly but recording was limited to two diagnoses for each patient in this study. Stroke was by far the commonest diagnosis, being present in about a quarter of admissions and discharges. The other common diagnoses were arthritis, fractured femur, balance problems and confusion—each being present in 8 to 9 per cent of cases.

It is noteworthy that 22 per cent of patients admitted had acute medical problems, suggesting that rehabilitation wards were being used for active medical management as well as the more traditional sub-acute and chronic disorders. Since so few patients were admitted directly from the accident and emergency departments to rehabilitation wards it is unlikely that this high level of acute problems was related to emergency admissions. Probably the acute condition was responsible for a decrease in mobility and function which required admission to a rehabilitation ward. It was obvious from talking to geriatricians that although some wards were designated primarily for rehabilitation there was a degree of flexibility linked to the pressure on the acute wards. Some geriatricians felt that a patient recently discharged from a rehabilitation ward who required readmission for an acute problem should be admitted to the original rehabilitation ward where the patient and staff knew each other.

The general impression gained was that there was a great deal of flexibility, even though wards were designated for rehabilitation or, for that matter, acute assessment. This has important implications for medical staffing and suggests that rehabilitation wards are suitable for training senior house officers and require supervision at registrar or senior registrar grade.

Table 18 Diagnoses of admissions and discharges on rehabilitation wards

Diagnosis	Admissions n=387 %	Discharges n=326 %	Total n=713 %
Neurological			
Stroke	27	20	24
Parkinsonism	3	5	4
Myopathy/neuropathy	2	2	2
'Cerebrovascular disease'	2	5	3
Balance problems	9	6	8
Mental			
Confusion	11	7	9
Depression	2	<1	2
Joint and bone			
Arthritis	10	9	9
Fractured femur	11	4	8
Other fracture	2	1	2
Spinal pain	2	2	2
Vascular			
Periph vasc disease	1	2	1
Amputation	2	2	2
Skin ulceration	4	2	3
Post-surgery	1	<1	1
General			
Carcinoma	1	4	2
'General frailty'	5	2	4
Incontinence	5	1	3
Acute			
Respiratory system	4	2	3
Myocardial infarction	1	1	1
Heart failure	8	9	8
'Acute medical'	9	15	11

Length of stay

Rehabilitation of the elderly is usually regarded as being a slow process. The second study showed the average length of stay on rehabilitation wards to be about 43 days, and approximately the same for males and females. However, about one third were either discharged or died within the first two weeks of admission, while 18 per cent had been in the rehabilitation ward for longer than two months and eight per cent for longer than four months (Table 19).

Prolonged length of stay was usually due to the waiting time for long-term residential care (Table 20). The shortest length of stay was for those who returned home—on average within about one month. Patients transferred to private rest or nursing homes were discharged, on average, about two weeks earlier than those transferred to social service homes, although it has to be recognised

Table 19 Length of stay of patients discharged from rehabilitation wards

	Male n=110 %	Female n=216 %	Total n=326 %
Length of stay (weeks)			
<2	36	28	31
−4	22	25	24
−8	20	27	25
−12	8	6	7
−16	3	4	3
≥16	9	7	8
Not stated	2	2	2
Mean (days)	41.1	43.9	43.0

that these patients may have had different degrees of disability and were therefore not necessarily comparable. On average, patients remained on the rehabilitation wards for about three months before being transferred to the long-stay wards.

Within these groups there was a very wide variation, as can be seen from Table 20. One third of those who returned home or died had a very short length of stay—less than one month. Only 5 per cent of those who eventually returned home were on the rehabilitation ward for longer than 14 weeks, while this time was exceeded

Table 20 Placement of discharged rehabilitation patients

Length of stay (weeks)	Home n=225 (69%) %	Part III* n=30 (9%) %	Private rest/ nursing home n=10 (3%) %	Long-stay n=12 (3%) %	Died n=39 (12%) %
<4	37	7	20	0	35
−6	27	17	30	20	22
−8	17	24	20	30	11
−10	9	3	10	10	5
−14	6	17	0	10	11
−18	2	14	0	0	8
>18	3	17	20	30	19
Mean length of stay (days)	31.4	70.8	56.1	81.7	70.2
Mean age (yrs)	78.9	82.5	74.3	83.1	80.1

*Social services residential home

by 31 per cent of those transferred to social service homes, 20 per cent of those going to private residential homes and 30 per cent transferred to long-stay wards. This may indicate the amount of rehabilitation time used to make patients 'fit' for residential care or may simply indicate the waiting time for long-term care. It is to be expected that the greater the disability the longer the rehabilitation period. For instance, in an earlier study[4] we found that stroke patients making the least recovery received the longest therapy time.

About 70 per cent of patients returned to their previous accommodation. As many as 12 per cent died on rehabilitation wards. Only 3 per cent required transfer to a long-stay ward, although 12 per cent were discharged to residential care, either in a social service or a private rest or nursing home. The very small proportion of patients transferred to long-stay care could be due to careful selection of patients, although it has to be remembered that 12 per cent died on the rehabilitation wards, suggesting that selection was not limited to those most likely to be discharged. It may simply indicate that rehabilitation wards often helped the patient to achieve the level of ability required for institutional care in either a social service residential home or a private rest home.

Follow-up arrangements

There are a number of possible organisational approaches to follow-up of elderly patients after discharge (Table 21). Men and women had similar patterns of follow-up: about one third were referred back to the general practitioner for management, a quarter continued their rehabilitation in a day hospital and one sixth were seen in the outpatient department. Thus the geriatrician continued to manage 44 per cent of those discharged. Day centres, as opposed to day hospitals, were very rarely used. This may indicate the type of

Table 21 Follow-up arrangements for patients discharged from rehabilitation wards

Number	Males 110	Females 216	Total 326
Follow-up	%	%	%
No follow-up	26	35	32
Outpatient clinic	15	18	17
Day hospital	32	25	27
Day centre	0	<1	<1
Domiciliary physio	1	0	<1
Relief admissions	7	6	6
Other speciality	0	1	1
Not applicable (died or long-stay)	19	15	17
Not stated	0	<1	<1

patient discharged from the units or the general lack of or waiting times for day centres. Some indication of the chronicity of the disorders treated on rehabilitation wards is that 6 per cent of the patients were followed up by regular relief admissions.

Patients discharged home were more likely to continue their treatment in the day hospital while those discharged to residential care were either not followed up or were seen in the outpatient department. No doubt the needs of the two groups are different. People discharged to residential homes are likely to have been more dependent and to have achieved the appropriate goals while they were in hospital. Those returning home are likely to have different long-term goals which will need to be modified as the patient adapts to life at home. The day hospital therefore acts as a halfway house, with a monitoring as well as a rehabilitation role.

Teaching

Education of medical, nursing and paramedical staff is an important role of the geriatric unit. Undergraduate and postgraduate medical teaching took place at one fifth of the rehabilitation units (Table 22). A similar proportion of units taught nurses in training and 13 per cent had post-basic nurse teaching sessions on the rehabilitation wards. Few units taught other paramedical staff. There is clearly

Table 22 Teaching on rehabilitation wards

Type of teaching	Wards involved (%)
Medical—undergraduate	22
Medical—postgraduate	19
Nurse—basic training	20
Nurse—post basic training	13
General practitioner	2
Multidisciplinary	2

more scope for professional education on rehabilitation wards. They offer excellent opportunities for training, including the concept of the team approach and an emphasis on the interaction between physical, mental, emotional and social factors.

Discussion

Although some units designate certain wards for rehabilitation there is great flexibility in their use; many patients with acute illnesses are also admitted. Few are admitted directly to rehabilitation wards from the accient and emergency department, but many are transferred from medical and surgical units. The special emphasis on stroke and fracture of the femur highlights the part that geriatric units have to play in neurological and orthopaedic rehabilitation and the importance of good working relationships between the geriatric unit and the orthopaedic and medical departments.

The advanced age of the patients treated on geriatric rehabilitation units is an indication of the difficulties likely to be faced in the future as the number of the very old increases. This needs to be taken into consideration when planning future services.

The multidisciplinary approach and the emphasis on the interaction of medical, psychological and social factors offer excellent opportunities for training all types of health professionals in good patient management.

4 Long-term care

Introduction

To some people geriatrics is synonymous with long-term care. There is no doubt that the specialty of geriatric medicine has grown out of the neglect in times past of elderly and disabled patients who lingered in chronic sick wards and workhouse infirmaries, in some cases for years at a time, without proper medical care. As has been traced in Chapter 1, the evolution of geriatric medicine centred first on attempts to rehabilitate many of these unfortunate people who were in the long stay-wards inherited by the first geriatricians. The next endeavour was to ensure, as far as possible, that patients were not transferred for long-term care until they had had full medical diagnosis and treatment and an opportunity for rehabilitation. Over the years, therefore, there has been a change of emphasis in geriatric medicine towards rehabilitation and acute care and assessment. However, the challenge of long-term care remains firmly with the geriatrician, and the management of patients in long-term care wards is as much his responsibility as is the assessment and rehabilitation that precedes their transfer.

With increasing emphasis on the acute side of geriatric medicine there may be a danger that the long-stay side will be neglected. In our studies we have therefore done two main things: first we have attempted to describe the disposition of long-stay patients in different geriatric departments and have given statistics about their age, sex, diagnosis and source of admission; second, we visited 36 different geriatric departments to try to assess the quality of long-term care in typical departments throughout the land.

It will be shown later (Table 30) that separate long-term care wards existed in 62 per cent of the departments in the UK (that is, those practising the AR/L system and the A/R/L system). In the remaining 38 per cent the long-stay patients were combined in wards with other types of patients, either rehabilitation or acute. In our second study we obtained information over a two-week period from 43 different departments with separate long-stay wards. During that time there was an average of 0.04 admissions per bed, equivalent to 0.78 admissions per bed in one year or an average stay of 468 days. The sources of admission of the 230 patients involved are shown in Table 23, together with comparable figures from the 36 units visited

Long-term care

in the fifth study. While there is broad agreement in these two studies, there are some definite differences. The main difference is in the number of admissions directly from the community: 16 per cent in study 2 and almost twice as many in study 5. Both figures are surprising, and the larger more so. If separate long-term care wards are part of a system of progressive patient care then it might have been imagined that only a very small proportion of patients would be admitted directly from the community. However, it is likely that many of them had been inpatients in the geriatric department and were fully assessed and rehabilitated, but, for one reason or another, their discharge home was unsuccessful. This was an assumption, since these facts are not obtainable from our information. It is likely also that a proportion of patients in long-stay wards are admitted as holiday breaks, planned readmissions (perhaps on a six weeks in, six weeks out basis) or as respite admissions.

Allowing for this difference between the two studies, the trend in the other figures is very much the same and indicates that over half the patients in geriatric long-stay wards have passed through the rest of the geriatric department, and more than 15 per cent have come from other hospital wards. Our visits showed that such transfers included 8 per cent from medical wards, 4.3 per cent from orthopaedic wards and 2.3 per cent from surgery or psychiatry.

Table 23   Admissions to long-stay wards

	Study 2 (2-week period)	Study 5 (visits to 36 units)
Admissions from	(n = 230)	(n = 785)
Geriatric wards	59%	52%
Other wards	19%	15%
Community (home or residential home)	16%	30%
Other hospitals	5%	1%
Not stated	1%	2%

Information on the outcome of patients in long-stay wards was obtained during the two-week period of study 2 when 199 patients were discharged, transferred or died. In fact, 81 per cent died and 4.5 per cent were transferred to other hospital wards, presumably for surgery or other acute treatment. Of the 14.5 per cent who were discharged, 5 per cent went to residential homes or private nursing homes. Therefore, about 10 per cent went home, but again a proportion of these may be on prearranged, intermittent or respite admissions.

The median length of stay for all patients in long-stay wards (Table 33) is 785 days. The age and sex distribution of this group is shown in Table 24 which indicates a very much longer stay for women and a longer stay as age progresses in those over 65. The range of length of stay is enormous, being well in excess of ten years for a small group of patients. The median is longest for the eight female patients under 65 (1450 days—almost four years); the maximum is 8039 days, or 22 years.

The difference in median length of stay according to the main diagnosis is shown in Table 25. The four major diagnostic groups are stroke, Parkinsonism, osteo-arthritis and fracture of the femur. Of these, stroke is far and away the most common, with a median length of stay of 480 days. Amputees have a relatively short stay (median 112), whereas the few patients with rheumatoid arthritis and heart disease have the longest stay of all.

Table 24 Median length of stay (days) on long-stay wards by age and sex

	Male		Female	
	n	median	n	median
<65	10	480	8	1450
65–74	68	267	64	463
75–84	82	301	257	468
85+	32	393	264	575

Table 25 Median length of stay (days) on long-stay wards by main diagnosis

	n	Median length of stay
Amputation	17	112
Cancer	14	169
COAD	6	240
Fractured femur	57	386
Parkinsonism	133	469
Stroke	602	480
OA	65	553
RA	16	769
Heart disease	7	871

Waiting lists for long-stay beds existed in almost half of the departments with separately designated beds. This, of course, excluded the five ARL departments. Of the remaining thirty-one, fourteen had no waiting list and seventeen had. They varied from around two weeks to longer than six months (in three of the departments).

Medical involvement

What is the physician's role in relation to geriatric long-term care? There can be no doubt that his first responsibility is to ensure that patients admitted to his long-stay beds are in need of long-term hospital care and that they have been fully investigated and given every opportunity for rehabilitation and resettlement, either in their own homes or in residential care. Having discharged that responsibility, the consultant must also ensure that appropriate day-to-day medical cover is available for patients who develop episodes of acute intercurrent illness. It is unlikely that the consultant will provide day-to-day cover (in fact, our study of 132 long-stay wards disclosed only 1 per cent in which the consultant did so: Table 26). As this table shows, responsibility is equally divided between junior hospital staff (principally senior house officers) and medical staff who are not in the training grades (general practitioner clinical assistants, hospital practitioners or associate specialists).

Table 26 Day-to-day responsibility on long-stay wards (n = 132)

House officer	3	(2%)
Senior house officer	61	(46%)
Registrar	2	(2%)
Others (hospital practitioner, clinical assistant, associate specialist)	66	(50%)
Consultant	1	(1%)

The consultant geriatrician, however, has the ultimate responsibility for all patients in his long-stay wards and it is up to him to organise their care to ensure two main objectives: firstly that while the patients are living in the wards they maintain optimal health and independence, and secondly that their quality of life in the wards is good. In regard to the first objective, the consultant should regularly review such overall problems as incontinence rates, the provision of wheelchairs and other equipment (and their state of repair) and the rate of falls and pressure sores. He should ensure that the medication for each patient is regularly reviewed and that, apart from the episodic care which may be given by other members of the staff, their whole medical condition is reviewed from time to time. As regards quality of life, most—but not all—consultants will acknowledge that this is their ultimate responsibility. Again it will hardly be their responsibility on a day-to-day basis, but they will be expected to give a lead, to suggest innovations and to encourage and facilitate the work of others. It is apparent that nurses and volunteer organisers are becoming much more involved in this aspect of long-term care, as are, to a much lesser extent, occupational therapists.

Perhaps the ultimate expression so far of the nurses' wish to assume a higher profile in this role is seen in the development of the three prototype NHS nursing homes. These are outside the purlieu of the geriatric service and the responsibility for overall direction and management, and for day-to-day care, lies with the nurse in charge. Medical care, when it is required, is requested episodically from the patient's general practitioner. However, the role of these nursing homes has yet to be assessed; they form an ongoing pilot study.

Consultant geriatricians therefore still retain an inescapable responsibility for the quality of care in their long-stay wards. With these considerations in mind it is interesting to view the extent to which consultants and other medical staff are involved. Tables 27 and 28 (derived from study 2) show these findings. The time per week spent by medical staff in long-stay wards is shown in Table 27.

Table 27   Time spent per week by medical staff in long-stay wards

		Number of units = 43	
	n (% of departments)	Mean no mins per bed	Mean no hours per 20-bed ward
Consultant	43 (100)	2.22	0.7
Senior registrar	10 (23)	1.56	0.5
Registrar	10 (23)	1.26	0.4
Senior house officer	23 (54)	3.42	1.1
House officer	4 (9)	2.88	1.0
Hospital practitioner	43 (100)	6.48	2.2
Total doctors	43 (100)	9.54	3.2

All 43 departments providing information had consultant involvement and also had involvement by staff in the non-training grades—mainly general practitioners on a sessional basis. In fact, non-training grades spent most time in long-stay wards—an average of 2.2 hours weekly in a twenty-bedded ward. This compares with 1.1 hours a week by senior house officers, who were involved in day-to-day care in just over half of the departments. Consultants spent less than one hour per week in a twenty-bedded ward.

Table 28 shows the frequency of consultant ward rounds which occur weekly in 59 per cent of the departments, fortnightly in 15 per cent and at greater intervals in 17 per cent. It is clear therefore that while consultants visit their long-stay wards every one or two weeks in the main, they do not spend very much time there.

Quality of life

During the visits to the 36 departments (study 5) information was obtained about the facilities available for the promotion of recreation and activities for long-stay patients and some estimate made about the extent of these facilities. In Table 29, departments with one or more long-stay wards are compared with those in which long-

Long-term care

Table 28 Frequency of consultant ward rounds in long-stay wards

Number of consultants	54	
More than once a week	7%	
Weekly	59%	66% weekly or more often
Fortnightly	15%	
Three-weekly	2%	28% every 2 to 4 weeks
Monthly	11%	
Less than monthly	4%	
Not stated	2%	

stay patients were in wards with other patients. Overall, recreational activities were estimated to be at a high level in 25 per cent of the departments and at a low level in another 25 per cent; the remaining 50 per cent had some activities, but not many. Only 11 per cent had activities organisers or a patients' committee and 25 per cent a special recreation room. Except for the recreation room, facilities were better in the departments with separate long-term care wards, although it is clear that in all of them the facilities lag far behind those which were provided in the most active departments.

An example of high level activity is in a large department with 140 long-stay beds situated in a general hospital. It has a specially adapted recreation room which includes an art studio, a quiet room and a large general purpose room. There is also a tea bar at a height suitable for patients in wheelchairs. A full-time organiser (paid as an occupational therapy aide) has devised a programme in cooperation with a full-time music therapist, a number of local authority adult education teachers and a large number of volunteers. Patients come down from the long-stay wards for morning or afternoon sessions (about 60–70 patients each day). There are small classes (with fifteen patients each) for painting, clay modelling, cooking, debating and music appreciation. In addition there are friendship clubs

Table 29 Activities and resources for long-stay patients with and without separate accommodation

	Separate long-stay accommodation?		
	Yes *(A/R/L + AR/L)*	No *(A/RL + ARL + mixed)*	Total
Activities + +	7 (32)*	2 (14)	9 (25)
Activities –	4 (18)	5 (36)	9 (25)
Activities organiser	3 (14)	1 (7)	4 (11)
Recreation room	5 (23)	4 (24)	9 (25)
Patients committee	3 (14)	1 (7)	4 (11)
Total units	22 (100)	14 (100)	36 (100)

*( ) = %

each day where patients from different wards meet for tea and social activities, including entertainment and games. Some of the long-stay patients have formed a choir and others a small percussion band, and together they perform concerts for the staff of the hospital and other patients, and for visiting groups. The staff and volunteers of this unit have been brave enough to organise a visit to Lourdes for fifteen of the long-stay patients. They were accompanied by twenty-five relatives, members of staff and volunteers, and all paid for themselves. Despite the profound disabilities of the patients they travelled on a regular commercial flight and spent three happy days living in a hotel and taking part in the activities at Lourdes. Now the staff and volunteers are raising money to buy a small country cottage where the long-stay patients will spend a few days at a time. They will go in small numbers and be accompanied by staff and volunteers.

In one or two departments a 'pub' has been developed in a day room as a focus for social activities. Departments have art classes, handicrafts, concerts, parties and visits to shops, pubs and places of interest, organised principally by nurses and occupational therapy helpers with the assistance of volunteers. The four units with fully employed activities organisers had the greatest scope for recreational facilities. (Figure 3 shows a sample activities timetable.)

Figure 3 Sample recreation unit activities programme

Staff	*Adult education teachers (■)*
Activities organiser	Art
Music therapist (†)	Cookery
Asst activities organisers (▲)	Handicrafts
Recreation unit nurse (●)	Pottery
Recreation unit nurse (*)	Tai chi
Volunteer recreation unit secretary	

Monday am	*Tuesday am*	*Wednesday am*	*Thursday am*	*Friday am*
Sing-along (*†)	Darts club (▲)	Friendship club (▲*)	Games club (▲*)	Friendship club (▲*)
Oak ward visit (●)	Tai chi (■*)	Band (†)	Music group (†) (Cedar/Oak— alternate weeks)	Handicrafts (■●)
	Holly ward visit (●)	Cedar ward visit (●)	Handicrafts (■●)	

Lunch break

Monday pm	*Tuesday pm*	*Wednesday pm*	*Thursday pm*	*Friday pm*
Classical music (†)	Special events (●▲)	Debating society (●▲)	Choir (▲†)	Art (*)
Beauty group (●▲)	(Crafts)	Classical music (†)	Cookery (●)	Cookery
Pottery (■*)	Pottery (■*)	Art (■*)	Recall session (*) (●)	Office duties (▲)
			Sister Maria (Thought for week)	

Unhappily, at the other end of the spectrum there were departments in which all long-stay patients were in geriatric chairs in their nightclothes, sitting beside their beds. In one or two departments a high proportion of beds with cot sides was noted.

Discussion

The question of whether old people needing long-term care in hospital are better provided for in special wards by themselves or in mixed wards (along with other patients, acutely ill or undergoing rehabilitation) will also be touched on in Chapter 5. There it will be shown that units with separate long-stay wards did not have a poorer discharge rate than those with mixed wards—indeed the opposite was the case. If discharge rate is regarded as a measure of effectiveness, the presence of separate long-stay wards is no disadvantage. It is well recognised, however, that the discharge rate is not the optimal measure of the quality of a geriatric service. Many other factors have to be taken into consideration although, unfortunately, most are not susceptible to measurement in the way that the discharge rate is. However, high among the measures of effectiveness must be quality of care and the data presented in this chapter give some measure of this. It must be said, however, that the quality of long-term care in the majority of geriatric departments of all types is still far too low. Only 25 per cent have separate recreation rooms and a good level of recreation activities for the patients, and only 11 per cent have activities organisers. Using these measures, however, we show (Table 29) that the proportion of departments with a good level of activities and an activities organiser or patients' committee is twice as great in those units which have separate long-stay wards.

One question is whether nurses, therapists or some other person should have responsibility for promoting recreational activities. From our observations on visits to the 36 departments we believe strongly that the quality of life of long-stay patients is much enhanced in departments with an activities organiser. On the whole, occupational therapists have limited interest in recreational work, although they say that they would like to be more involved in work in long-stay wards if they had more staff (see Chapter 7). Nurses are also very ambivalent about their involvement in recreational activities in long-stay wards. In exceptional cases they are extremely active. A serious problem for activities organisers is that there is no career grade for them in the NHS at present. In the USA they have a proper training and administrative structure and it seems essential that the UK should move towards this. With the emergence of large numbers of private nursing homes offering long-term care, it is now a matter of particular urgency. The proper development of recreational activities should be seen as an essential part of their programme, just as it should be in geriatric wards.

It would seem from our studies that consultant geriatricians take their role seriously in relation to long-stay patients. Sixty per cent visit their long-stay wards every week and spend an average of over an hour per week to a twenty-bedded ward. However, a small proportion (15 per cent) visit only monthly, or even less often.

Another aspect of long-term care which is subject to criticism is the fact that they have fewer student nurses than other types of wards (see Chapter 6). Only 10 per cent of the staff on long-stay wards are learners compared with 27 per cent on acute wards and 33 per cent on mixed acute and rehabilitation wards. It is argued in Chapter 6 that there is more justification for training student nurses on long-stay than on acute geriatric wards since acute wards are little different from acute medical wards. Long-term care, on the other hand, provides a very special field of nursing which is entirely different and, in its widest sense (including psychiatry, psychogeriatrics and mental subnormality), involves a larger proportion of hospital beds within the NHS than the acute specialties.

The final conclusion from this chapter, therefore, is that long-term care provides a unique form of geriatric practice requiring the committed involvement of consultants, the appointment of activities organisers and the training of student nurses. Even if there is a move away from providing long-term care in geriatric units towards NHS and private nursing homes, these considerations will still apply if this form of geriatric practice is to receive its rightful and necessary recognition.

5 Variations in the style of geriatric practice

Introduction

While the essence of the practice of geriatric medicine consists of the basic ingredients of acute medicine, rehabilitation and long-term care, together with the day hospital and community involvement, the ways in which these different elements are welded together in a geriatric unit vary widely. They derive in part from the history of the department, in part from the disposition of its resources, and in part from the philosophy of the consultant or consultants most involved in establishing it. Some departments have all their beds on one site and serve a dense population in a relatively small area. Others may have beds in four, five or six different hospitals perhaps spread over a rural area of hundreds of square miles. Some have developed in hospitals where there has been a shortage of general medical or psychiatric facilities and may therefore have tended to lay more emphasis on these elements in geriatric practice. Others may have inherited a tradition of receiving most of their patients from other clinicians and found it difficult to establish their own direct admissions. The pioneers of age-related policies such as those in Oldham[1] and Hull[2] found it most advantageous to admit acutely ill patients to every ward, where they shared accommodation with patients undergoing rehabilitation and those needing long-term care. Others insisted on the use of separate wards for these three functions.

In fact there are three major patterns which cover 83 per cent of units in the country according to our first study (Table 30)*. The most common—38 per cent—combines acute and rehabilitation patients in one group of wards and has separate wards for long-stay patients. The next most common, 24 per cent, comprises the traditional progressive patient care system with separate acute, rehabilitation and long-stay wards. The third, 21 per cent, combines acute, rehabilitation and long-term patients in each ward. These three patterns, together with the small proportion of others, are shown in Table 30. It follows from these figures that separately designated acute geriatric wards may be expected in 24 per cent of

---

*Tables 30, 34, 36, 37 and 38 are reproduced from *Age and Ageing* 1984, 14, pages 3–5, with permission of the publishers.

Table 30 Styles of geriatric units in the UK

Design	Number	%
AR/L	80	38
A/R/L	52	24
ARL	45	21
A/RL	16	8
RL	5	2
Combinations	15	7

departments, separate rehabilitation wards in 24 per cent and separate long-stay wards in 62 per cent. Combined rehabilitation and long-stay wards (with no designated acute beds) comprise only 2 per cent.

If these labels truly indicate different styles of practice, the different types of ward should be quite dissimilar in their sources of admission and in the length of stay of their patients. Tables 31, 32 and 33, derived from the second study, describe a cross section of patients in these different types of ward at any one time. Table 31 shows the proportions admitted to the different types of ward directly from the community, either through accident and emergency or by arrangement with the general practitioner from their own homes or from residential homes. As might be expected, such

Table 31 Sources of admission to different types of ward

	a) Admissions from the community (%) (n = 1250)			
	Via accident & emergency department	Home	Residential home	Total from the community
A	7.8	77.4	6.1	91.3
R	0.8	37.1	5.8	43.7
AR	1.0	73.4	4.8	79.2
ARL	8.0	65.0	6.4	79.4
RL	4.3	39.8	8.1	52.2
L	0	23.6	6.1	29.7

admissions comprise over 90 per cent of patients in acute wards and almost 80 per cent of those in A/R and ARL wards. It is surprising, however, that 44 per cent of patients admitted to rehabilitation wards and 52 per cent admitted to RL wards have also come directly from the community. It suggests that in many wards facilities for acute medical work-up must be available. If this is the case it would have implications for medical staffing which will be considered later. Almost 30 per cent of patients admitted to long-stay wards also come directly from the community and it may well be that many of them have previously been inpatients in other wards and further

Variations in the style of geriatric practice

acute or rehabilitation intervention was not thought necessary. It is also likely that in all wards, other than acute, a proportion of admissions will be intermittent or respite admissions—patients admitted for short periods on regular occasions according to a pre-arranged plan. These admissions are to help carers by giving them a break from time to time—a respite they know they can depend on.

Table 32 shows the proportion of patients transferred to different types of geriatric ward from other hospital wards. As might be expected, they comprise more than two thirds of the patients transferred to long-stay wards. About half of long-stay admissions are transferred from other parts of the geriatric department. It is also to be expected that a high proportion of patients admitted to rehabilitation wards will be transfers; in fact, 30 per cent came from geriatric wards and 25 per cent from other wards. The 11.3 per cent from medical wards may be expected to comprise largely stroke patients and those from other wards (orthopaedic and surgical) with femoral fracture or leg amputation.

Table 32 Sources of admission to different types of ward

	b) Intra-hospital transfers (%)				
	Geriatric ward	*Medical ward*	*Other ward*	*Other hospital*	*Total hospital transfers*
A	0.8	3.9	3.4	0.6	8.7
R	30.8	11.3	13.3	0.4	55.8
AR	5.2	6.2	6.2	3.1	20.7
ARL	5.5	4.0	8.0	1.8	19.3
RL	16.1	1.6	8.0	1.1	26.8
L	51.6	8.0	6.6	1.4	67.6

The median length of stay in different types of wards is shown in Table 33. As might be expected, it is 14 days in acute wards, 29 days in rehabilitation wards and 475 days in long-stay wards. The range, of course, is enormous and the extreme of 8000 days and more—a length of stay of over 22 years—must be grossly exceptional and, hopefully, will not be repeated in the future.

When the different types of unit are examined individually it is apparent that there is some overall variation in turnover of patients (Table 34, derived from the first study). Patient turnover may be judged from the mean number of discharges per bed per year, which is highest in the A/R/L units and lowest in the AR/L units. The number of discharges per population (1000 persons aged 65 and over in the catchment area) per year shows little variation however (from 36.6 in AR/L to 42.6 in A/R/L). These figures suggest that

Table 33 Length of stay in different types of geriatric wards

	No of patients	Median length of stay (days)	Range (days)
A	358	14	1–1266
R	240	29	1–3426
AR	289	43	1–2751
ARL	326	49	1–5974
RL	186	159	1–4954
L	785	475	1–8039

Table 34 Type of service compared with resources and discharge rate

		AR/L	A/R/L	ARL	A/RL	Significance
Beds/	Mean	9.55	8.66	8.06	7.94	AR/L v ARL
population	SEM	0.36	0.39	1.42	0.47	t = 2.650 df121; p<0.01
Beds/	Mean	140.88	125.67	120.30	140.42	AR/L v ARL
consultant	SEM	6.30	5.53	6.86	15.85	t = 2.089 df121; p<0.05
Discharges/	Mean	3.93	5.21	4.97	4.92	AR/L v A/R/L p<0.02*
bed/year						AR/L v ARL p<0.025
Discharges/	Mean	34.62	42.62	38.16	40.29	AR/L v A/R/L p<0.05*
population						
Long-stay/ total beds (estimated)	Mean	59.58	52.92	50.48	43.78	

*Mann-Whitney

bed provision varies in the different types of unit. This is borne out in part from the figures shown in Table 35 which indicate that the AR/L units have the highest average number of beds per population. The lowest however are shared by the A/RL and the ARL units. There is also a variation in the number of beds looked after by an individual consultant, and this difference is significant in comparing ARL units (where a consultant has care of an average of 120 beds) with AR/L units (where the figure is 141). Otherwise, there are no great differences in the staffing resources of the different types of service except for social workers, where again the combined ARL units are significantly better off than the AR/L units (Table 36).

Since we are dealing with mean figures for a very large number of departments (193 altogether) it is reasonable to expect some

Variations in the style of geriatric practice

relationship between the different types of department and these findings. Such a relationship may be derived from the different types of geographical area in which departments are situated, or from the way in which consultants practise in different types of unit. Possibly,

Table 35 Resources in different types of geriatric units*

	Style of practice				
	A/R/L	AR/L	A/RL	ARL	UK
Beds/population					
No of units	52	79	15	43	207
Mean beds/pop	8.7	9.5	7.9	8.0	8.7
SEM	0.39	0.36	0.47	0.37	0.41
<6	14%	10%	20%	21%	15%
−7.5	21%	19%	7%	21%	20%
−9	35%	25%	40%	26%	29%
−10.5	15%	14%	27%	16%	15%
−13.5	6%	20%	7%	16%	15%
>13.5	10%	11%	0	0	7%
Consultants/population					
No of units	52	79	15	43	
Mean consultants/population	0.076	0.073	0.062	0.078	0.07
SEM	0.005	0.003	0.005	0.007	0.002
<0.04	12%	6%	7%	9%	9%
−0.08	54%	62%	74%	63%	61%
−0.12	27%	26%	20%	16%	23%
>0.12	8%	7%	0	12%	7%
Beds/consultant					
No of units	52	80	16	45	212
Beds/consultant	125.7	140.9	140.4	120.3	131.3
SEM	5.5	6.3	15.9	6.9	4.4
<100	38%	23%	31%	33%	30%
−160	40%	45%	38%	49%	45%
>160	21%	33%	31%	18%	25%
Beds/unit					
<150	15%	18%	25%	31%	22%
−250	35%	45%	38%	40%	38%
−350	23%	24%	19%	13%	20%
>350	27%	14%	19%	16%	20%
Population/unit					
<22,500	25%	41%	19%	31%	31%
−37,500	48%	38%	50%	40%	38%
>37,500	27%	21%	25%	19%	30%
Consultants/unit					
1	23%	35%	38%	31%	
2	42%	48%	44%	51%	
3	23%	14%	13%	4%	
>4	12%	4%	6%	13%	

Statistical significances are as follows:
Beds/pop   AR/L v ARL $t = 2.650$ df121 $p < .01$
Beds/consultant AR/L v ARL $t = 2.089$ df121 $p < .05$

*Excluding RL and mixed units

Table 36 Staff levels (mean values) in different types of geriatric units

Staffing ratio per population	AR/L	A/R/L	ARL	A/RL	Significance
Consultant	0.07	0.08	0.08	0.06	ns
Physiotherapist	0.14	0.15	0.16	0.15	ns
Occupational therapist	0.10	0.09	0.11	0.10	ns
Social workers	0.08	0.09	0.10	0.09	AR/L v ARL $p<0.02$*
Speech therapists	0.04	0.02	0.03	0.02	ns

*Mann-Whitney

there is an intrinsic difference between these styles of practice which brings about different discharge rates and different levels of staffing.

The comparison of the different types of areas with styles of practice is shown in Table 37. There are no significant differences here but there are some trends. In particular, the ARL units cluster more in the cities and the A/R/L in the large towns, where it may be easier to achieve higher staffing levels. The AR/L units on the other hand are more predominant in rural areas.

It would be hazardous from the data presented here to suggest that one style of practice is more effective than another. This is particularly the case in relation to discharge rates since it is well known that a high discharge rate may hide an equally high readmission rate. Also it says nothing for the quality of care given by the department. At the same time, discharge rate is one of the few measurable indices for comparing one department with another and the fact that progressive patient care units (A/R/L type) have the highest would at least tend to confirm that this style of practice does not use beds inefficiently. The argument that it is more effective to admit patients directly to any geriatric ward where a place is available is not borne out by these figures. This may be kept in mind when examining the function of the rehabilitation and long-stay components of these units in other chapters. Indeed, it might be argued that the A/R/L style offers greater scope for environmental control during the different stages in geriatric patient care, and therefore has much to offer as a model of management.

Table 37 Numbers of departments and types of service in different population groups (as percentages)

Type of service	% of total	City $n=33$	Mainly urban $n=30$	Urban/rural $n=43$	Mainly rural $n=85$	Coastal $n=10$	Academic $n=13$
A/R/L	24	18	40	26	20	20	31
AR/L	38	30	33	33	45	30	38
A/RL	8	12	7	7	6	20	38
ARL	21	27	20	21	19	10	31
Other	9	12	—	13	11	20	

Variations in the style of geriatric practice

Specialist services

A development in geriatric practice at the present time is the emergence of specialist services, such as those for stroke rehabilitation, and those offered by combined orthopaedic/geriatric units and the more widely developed psychogeriatric and younger-disabled units. Stroke rehabilitation and ortho-geriatric rehabilitation units are intrinsic to geriatric departments, whereas the others are generally separate and in most cases managed by other clinicians (psychiatrists in the case of psychogeriatrics; and neurologists, orthopaedic surgeons or rheumatologists in the case of younger-disabled units). Information on the provision of these types of service was obtained in study 1 from 213 of the 220 departments replying. The findings are in Table 38. There is not much variation in relation to style of practice but the small number of AR/L units

Table 38 **Special organisations associated with geriatric units**

	Style of practice				
	A/R/L	AR/L	A/RL	ARL	Total
Orthogeriatric unit	29%	14%	38%	16%	43
Stroke unit	17%	6%	13%	11%	23
Day hospital	96%	91%	94%	89%	178
Young-disabled unit	33%	31%	44%	33%	75
Domiciliary physiotherapy	75%	64%	44%	64%	143

share with the A/R/L units a higher proportion of orthopaedic/geriatric special units; A/R/L also have a higher proportion of stroke units and a higher availability of domiciliary physiotherapy. These figures may relate to the special interests developed by consultants working with separate rehabilitation wards.

Discussion

It may seem surprising that there is such variation in styles of practice in a specialty which has now been established for nearly 40 years. This must be due largely to the heterogeneous groups of hospitals which go to make up individual geriatric departments. For instance, in the 36 units visited as part of this study the numbers of hospitals in which geriatric beds were deployed are as follows:

8 hospitals in 2 departments
7 ,, ,, 2 ,,
5 ,, ,, 2 ,,
4 ,, ,, 10 ,,
3 ,, ,, 12 ,,
2 ,, ,, 8 ,,

The mean was 3.7 hospitals per department. In general, the style of practice does not seem to reflect geographical variations although there are some exceptions. Rural areas tend to have a higher percentage of combined acute and rehabilitation wards with separate long-stay wards, while urban areas tend to have a service based on separate acute, rehabilitation and long-stay wards. However, these are only trends.

The major difference in practice is whether acute emergencies are admitted to all geriatric wards (ARL) or whether there are separate acute wards (A/R/L and AR/L). This difference is associated with a difference in philosophy and applies especially to the departments which have separate long-stay wards (32 per cent have separate acute wards and 62 per cent separate long-stay wards).

The management of acute illness in the elderly differs in degree rather than in kind from the management of acute medical illness in younger people. The need is for a ward fitted for the care of medical emergencies in the elderly, with staff specially trained to manage them. Provision for long-term care is very different; the most important considerations are privacy, recreational activities and an environment and pace of life fit for old people, for whom the ward is home. Staff training and perceptions have to be very different and the ability to develop patients' and relatives' committees, to organise visits out of the hospital, and to foster a close and continuing relationship between patients and staff would seem to be extremely important. It could be argued that these are qualities difficult to provide in a ward where nurses also have to devote a good deal of their time to newly admitted patients with medical emergencies. Similarly, the processes of rehabilitation require a particular environment and the use of a rehabilitation team unsuited to either an acute ward or a long-stay ward.

Perhaps one important finding in this chapter is the fact that departments having separate acute, rehabilitation and long-stay wards do not, in consequence, have a lower turnover of patients. In fact, if discharge rate is a criterion of effectiveness, these types of wards, which on average have the highest discharge rate, might be deemed the most effective. It is generally appreciated that discharge rate may not be the best parameter of geriatric care and that what really matters is the quality of care offered and its appropriateness to the patients. This would seem to be best obtained in specialised separate wards catering for different needs.

6 Nurse provision

One of the greatest sources of controversy between clinicians and nurses on the one hand and managers and treasurers on the other, centres round the numbers of nurses required in geriatric wards. It might seem relatively simple to carry out a work study exercise to determine the exact nature of the tasks to be carried out, the best way of doing them, the times of day when they need to be done, and the time required over and above these tasks for communication with patients, relatives and others. In fact, it is extremely complex and so far no generally accepted formula has been reached, partly because of the enormous variations in style of practice as outlined earlier in this book, and partly because of the variability of the nursing environment, particularly ward architecture. Wells[1], for example, has described the problems inherent in both the architectural layout of different wards and in the nature of the equipment provided. Work studies might give staffing figures for the ideal ward design provided with all the necessary equipment. Since there is no consensus as to what is ideal in design or in equipment this goal is clearly unattainable. There can be little doubt that in the majority of geriatric wards, the layout is far from ideal and has evolved in buildings 50 to 100 years old, where bed numbers have gradually been diminished and day space introduced. A formula for ideal nurse staffing ratios would have to take these variables into account.

Staffing levels

In the personal visits made to 193 wards in 36 different hospitals, the numbers of nurses on duty on the day of the visit were noted for four times during the day—9.30am, 2.30pm, 7pm and the previous night. All nursing staff, including the charge nurse or sister and the auxiliaries were noted. Those nurses who were scheduled for duty but who were off sick or had been seconded to other wards were excluded. Other information collected in each ward included the number of beds, the number of patients (that is, the number of occupied beds) and the type of designation which the ward carried (acute, rehabilitation, and so on).

From these findings it has been possible to build up a profile of the numbers of nursing staff on duty in different types of ward and in different parts of the country. While these figures only describe the present situation and not the ideal, they do give a yardstick for comparison and also indicate the best staffed and the worst staffed ward types and geographical areas.

Table 39* shows the number of beds per nurse through different times of the day as well as the number of occupied beds per nurse. This indicates that 2.30pm is the time of best staffing when 4.3 beds per nurse or 4.0 occupied beds per nurse was the mean. The figures for the morning (4.8 and 4.3 respectively) were less advantageous and by 7pm each nurse had 6.9 beds or 6.4 patients to care for. The figures during the night, as might be expected, were even higher with 8.8 patients per nurse.

Table 39 also shows the figures by quintiles and this indicates (for instance for 9.30am) that the best staffed fifth of the wards had 2.4 beds per nurse, whereas the worst staffed fifth had 6.0 beds per nurse. At 2.30pm the comparison is even more striking between 1.7 and 6.3 beds per nurse. These figures show that there is a 200 per

Table 39 Beds per nurse at different times of the day

		Morning (9.30am)	Afternoon (2.30pm)	Evening (7pm)	Night
Total nurses		974	1054	659	477
Beds per nurse (mean)		4.8	4.3	6.9	10.3
Beds per nurse by quintiles	100%	2.4	1.7	3.4	5.3
	80%	4.0	3.4	6.0	8.0
	60%	4.6	4.2	6.7	9.8
	40%	5.2	5.0	7.5	10.5
	20%	6.0	6.3	8.7	12.5
Occupied beds per nurse (mean)		4.3	4.0	6.4	8.8

cent to 300 per cent difference between wards as to the nurse staffing ratios. The particularly large variation at 2.30pm is partly explained by the fact that some hospitals have an overlap of shifts at that time. These figures are shown graphically (on a logarithmic scale) in Figure 4.

Table 40 shows the variation in occupied beds per nurse in different types of ward and indicates that at all times the wards with long-stay patients (L) or with a mixture of rehabilitation and long-stay patients (RL), are the worst staffed. The total number of beds per nurse in the different kinds of wards during the morning is

---

*Tables 40, 41, 42 and 43 and Figures 4, 5 and 6 are reproduced by kind permission of *Nursing Times* where they first appeared in an Occasional Paper on February 4th, 1987.

Nurse provision

Figure 4 Ratio of beds per nurse (193 wards)

The figures are shown by quintiles; the dotted line represents the mean.

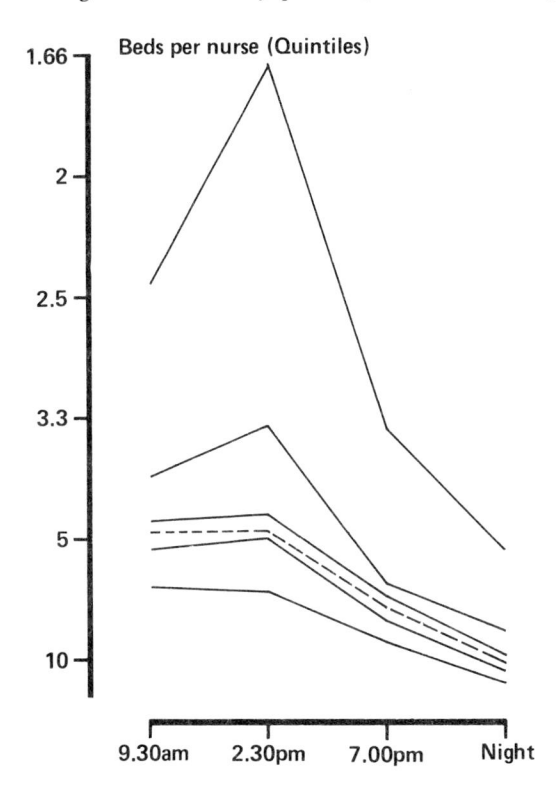

```
Beds per nurse (Quintiles)
1.66
2
2.5
3.3
5
10
      9.30am   2.30pm   7.00pm   Night
```

shown in Figure 5 by quintiles. This shows some differences in as much as the top 20 per cent of long-stay wards are better staffed than all others except the AR wards. However, this advantage does not hold for the other 80 per cent of the long-stay wards.

Table 41 shows the average percentage of learners in the different types of wards and the numbers of occupied beds per nurse if the learners are excluded. There is more than a threefold difference in the percentage of learners in different types of wards, the highest (33.1 per cent) being in combined acute and rehabilitation wards and the lowest (10.1 per cent and 10.2 per cent) in ARL and L wards respectively.

It is clear that acute geriatric wards are regarded as more suitable for training student nurses than are long-stay wards. This is a concept which might be challenged.

Table 42 shows the percentage of trained staff, untrained staff and learners in the different types of wards in the morning. The total

Figure 5 Beds per nurse, beds per trained nurse and percentage of beds occupied in different types of wards

The figures are shown by quintiles; the dotted line represents the mean.

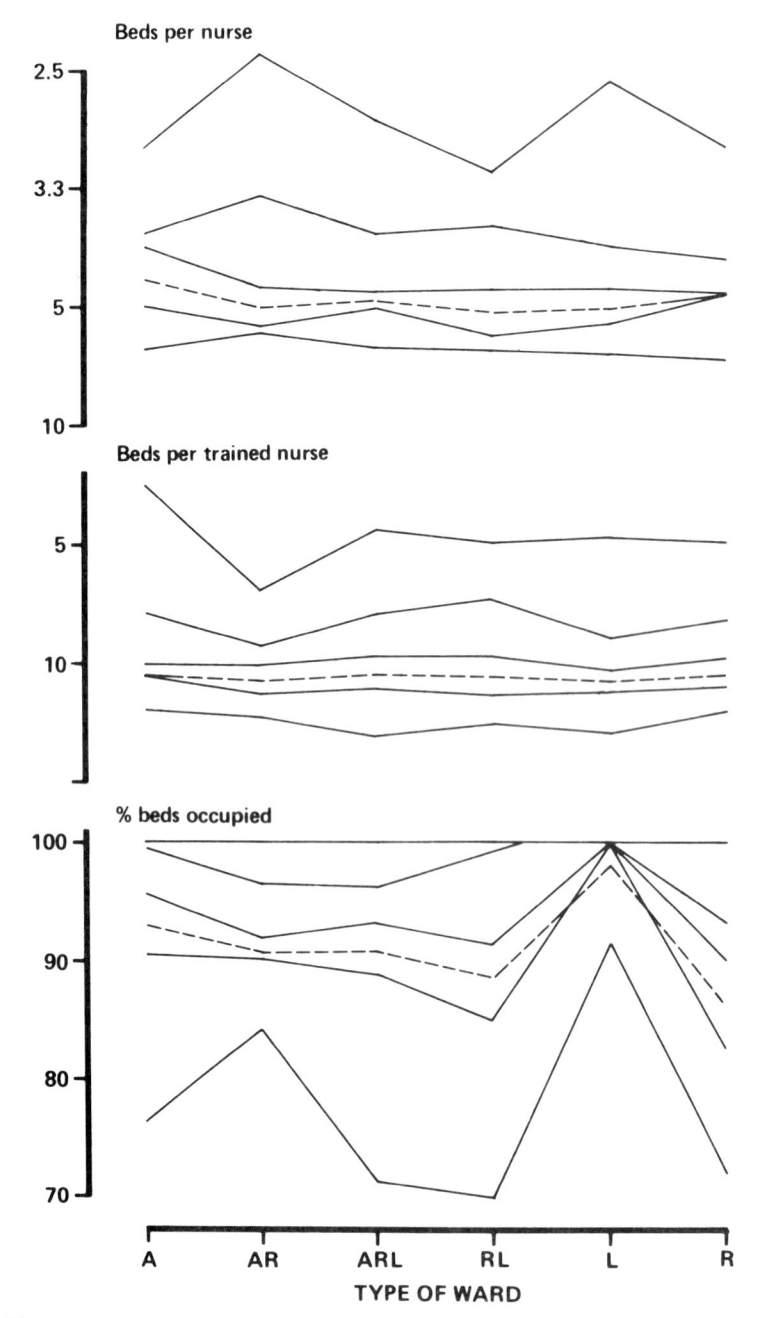

Nurse provision

Table 40 Occupied beds per nurse in different types of wards at various times throughout a 24-hour period (mean figure)

	Beds per nurse			
	Morning (9.30am)	Afternoon (2.30pm)	Evening (7pm)	Night
A	4.1	3.7	6.1	8.1
R	4.2	4.1	5.6	8.0
L	4.6	4.3	6.6	9.4
AR	4.0	3.1	6.3	8.6
RL	4.5	4.4	6.8	9.5
ARL	4.0	4.2	6.5	8.6
Total	4.3	4.0	6.4	8.8
Total nurses	974	1054	659	477

Table 41 Number of occupied beds and nurses on duty in different types of wards at 9.30am

Type of ward	No of wards	Occupied beds	No of nurses	% learners	Occupied beds/nurse excluding learners
A	36	760	186	26.9	6.3
R	21	391	94	20.9	6.2
L	66	1451	313	10.2	5.4
AR	20	500	124	33.1	6.6
RL	23	486	109	19.3	6.3
ARL	27	600	149	10.1	5.1
Total	193	4188	974	18.3	5.8

percentage of trained staff varies from 41 per cent in AR wards to 46 per cent in acute wards and rehabilitation wards. The proportion of untrained staff is highest in long-stay wards (48 per cent) and ARL wards (45 per cent). These figures are almost twice those for the acute wards (26 per cent). If the learners are omitted from the calculation then the percentage of trained staff is very much of a similar order comparing the different types of ward.

Table 43 shows the variation in percentage of trained staff at different times of day by quartiles. The figures do not vary greatly but show that in the later part of the day and at night the proportion of trained staff diminishes (12 per cent having more than half trained staff at night, compared with 28 per cent and 33 per cent having more than half trained staff at 9.30am and 2.30pm respectively).

The variation of staff by different geographical locality is shown in Figure 6 for 9.30am. This shows a strikingly higher proportion of unoccupied beds in small towns but no other real differences.

Table 42 Comparison of trained and untrained nurses and learners in different types of wards

Type of ward	% Nursing staff					
	SRN	SEN	Learners	Untrained	Total trained	% trained (omitting learners)
A	20	26	27	26	46	64
R	23	23	21	33	46	59
L	20	22	10	48	42	47
AR	15	26	33	26	41	62
RL	21	21	19	38	42	52
ARL	21	24	10	45	45	50
Total	20	24	18	38	44	54

(All figures to nearest whole number.)

Table 43 Trained nursing staff on duty at different times of day

	% Trained staff on duty at different times of the day, by quartiles			
Trained staff	9.30am	2.30pm	7.00pm	Night
<25%	20	14	19	15
26–50%	51	53	61	74
51–75%	25	26	15	7
>75%	3	7	6	5

(Figures represent % of 193 wards to nearest whole number.)

Discussion

The first question that has to be answered is whether these nurse staffing levels are those that are really required to look after geriatric patients. The second is whether it is reasonable that there should be such variation between the best served and the worst served wards, and the third concerns the position of the learners.

It has already been indicated that there are difficulties in laying down a standard norm in view of the considerable variation in facilities required and work that has to be done. However, this should not prevent us trying to make some attempt to define the factors that must be considered. A study carried out in 1966 by a joint working party of the Royal College of Nursing, the National Council of Nurses of the UK and The Hospital Centre[2] laid down a number of general principles in relation to nurse staffing in hospitals: 1) the need to assess the patient care required in each ward and department; 2) to plan to use every hour of nursing available as economically as possible by employing nurses at times when the workload is greatest; 3) to remember that student nurses do not give full-time nursing service to the patients; 4) to allow sufficient nurses to cover sickness, holidays and incidental staff

Nurse provision

Figure 6 Beds per nurse, beds per trained nurse and percentage of beds occupied in different types of geographical areas

The figures are shown by quintiles; the dotted line represents the mean.

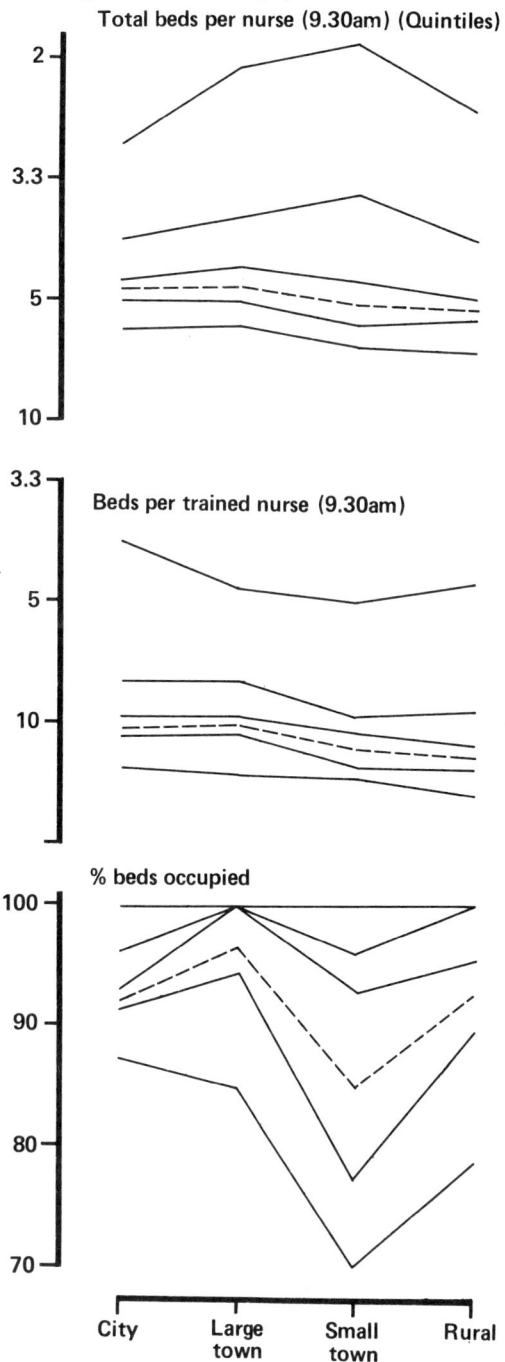

shortages. Among their other recommendations was the need to take into consideration the building and the architectural features which make for extravagance or economy in staffing. They also urge that the money supplied to pay for nursing staff not be reduced or frozen at short notice. The working party concluded:

'Just as patients are people, so are nurses. The quality of care that they give to their patients will depend largely on two factors—their own personal standards and integrity, and upon the tradition, atmosphere and morale that exists within the complex organism that is a hospital.'

Another striking and relevant quotation from the nursing literature on geriatric services in the UK states:

'The environments in which nursing care took place were not supportive and in some instances were impossible. The tools with which to give nursing care were most often inadequate, insufficient and substandard. The changes imposed upon nursing care, such as personalised clothing, were based on a lack of knowledge about current practice, lack of thoughtful planning and lack of evaluation. While untrained staff had little idea of cause and care of common problems of the elderly, the knowledge of trained staff was also vague, confused and inadequate. Moreover, nursing work routines created irrational and impossible work goals'[1].

From her detailed study, Wells concluded that the most important index of good nursing practice in geriatrics was the nurse-patient relationship and the way that this was expressed in communication. She found that nurses infrequently talked to patients and that when they did so, they were more concerned about tasks than about the patient as a thinking, feeling person. A further quotation sums up this view succinctly:

'Nurses are not taught how to develop effective and meaningful nurse-patient relationships. They are taught about tasks. Nurses do not receive any guidance on the development of relationships with patients in the clinical setting. Instead they are expected to get through the tasks and keep the ward tidy.'[1]

The conflict between task-orientated and patient-centred nursing is now widely discussed and great strides are being made in developing the latter through the nursing process. The benefits of individualised care (the nursing process) in geriatric patients have recently been convincingly demonstrated by Miller[3]. Those whose care was individualised were significantly less dependent, less apathetic and had fewer problems in communication than a comparable group whose nursing was task-orientated.

The principles and practice of primary nursing have been described in detail by McFarlane & Castledine[4]. They indicate that the primary nurse is responsible for the care of patients throughout their stay in hospital, assisted by a second or associate nurse who cares for the patient when the primary nurse is off duty. The primary nurse should be a trained nurse and the second nurse may be a learner or an auxiliary. Since it is not always possible to have these two nurses working on opposite shifts, all nurses on the ward must serve as associates for their colleagues. The primary nurse is responsible for assessing the patient's nursing needs and drawing up a care plan, working with the patient while on duty and serving as the main coordinator of the patient's total care. The primary nurse would present the case at nursing evaluation sessions and at ward rounds and may make home visits prior to, or following, discharge. It is suggested that the primary nurse's name is placed over each patient's bed. The sister/charge nurse should retain responsibility for the care plan of a few patients and delegate responsibility for others to her staff.

McFarlane and Castledine suggest a primary nurse:patient ratio in the region of 1:4 on day duty, depending on the type of care needed and the rapidity of patient turnover. The nurse:patient ratio in Miller's study, described above, was one trained nurse (or senior student nurse) as the primary nurse for six to eight patients, assisted by two auxiliaries or junior student nurses.

Can geriatric nursing care be provided with the staff ratios that have been described here? Unfortunately we cannot come to any firm conclusion about this from the figures presented here since, even if one takes the numbers of trained and untrained nurses on duty at different times of the day compared with the number of patients, this will not allow a calculation of the total number of trained nurses available to a ward. If all primary nurses are to be trained nurses then a 20-bed ward would require four trained nurses in order to allocate five patients to each of them. This recognises the fact that the primary nurse is likely to be on duty for less than one third of the total number of daytime hours in the week (if we take a twelve-hour day and a seven-day week). Thus, a high bed:nurse ratio does not necessarily exclude primary nursing. In fact, in the wards studied by Miller there was an average of seven trained nurses on the weekly duty rotas which (excluding the ward sister), in a 28-bed ward, meant an average of about five patients each. In the wards she studied which were using primary nursing, the mean number of beds per nurse at 9.30am was 5.37 (Miller, personal communication). Thus the changes she described in her paper were achieved with staffing ratios which were poorer than the mean throughout the country. It is her view that accountability rather than staffing levels produced the improved patient outcome.

A study of the nursing load involved in caring for geriatric patients was described by Magid and Rhys Hearn[5]. They recorded the dependency characteristics of 7561 patients comprising those in all geriatric wards in the West Midlands region and one ward in each district of the North West Thames region. Interestingly, they found that 59.7 per cent were long-stay patients and only 12.6 per cent were acute or assessment patients. The ratio of long-stay patients is higher, and of acute patients lower than is probably the case generally throughout the country, although we cannot quantify the types of patient from our study of 36 different health authorities since not every ward was sampled. Their findings, shown in Table 44, indicate an enormously high level of dependency. Some of these factors (for example, urinary and faecal incontinence) might be considerably diminished by better nursing care with larger numbers of nurses available. Among other items of special care undertaken on the day of the survey, they found that 13 per cent of patients either had suppositories or enemas, 12 per cent required blood pressure measurements and 12 per cent dressings. The level of technical nursing was less than 10 per cent of nursing time for the non-acute patients, but over 20 per cent for acute patients.

It is worth remembering that less than half of nursing auxiliaries on long-term wards have had any in-service training[6].

One well-known study which attempted to quantify nurse staffing requirements is that of the Scottish Home and Health Department[7].

Table 44   Dependency on nurses by geriatric patients

		%
Conscious level	Unconscious	1.1
Mobility	Bedfast/chairfast	7.2
	Mobile independently (aids or wheelchair)	32.0
	Mobile with nurse(s)	68.0
Continence Urine	Continent	31.0
	Sometimes incontinent	35.0
	Often/always incontinent	22.0
	Indwelling catheter	11.0
Continence Faeces	Continent	45.0
	Sometimes incontinent	37.0
	Often/always incontinent	17.0
	Colostomy	1.0
Self care	Requires assistance with:	
	Feeding	18.0
	Washing	62.0
	Dressing	55.0

Figures taken from Magid and Rhys Hearn's 1981 study of 7561 patients.

They categorised patients in terms of dependency. Most geriatric patients in long-stay wards would fall into their category B (bedfast/chairfast and partially helpless) or category C (bedfast/chairfast and not helpless). On this basis, assuming additional allowances for technical nursing, administrative duties, domestic work and miscellaneous duties, the figures for female geriatric long-stay wards work out at 17.1 hours per week for category B and 16.2 hours per week for category C. In a ward with ten patients in each category the workload per week is therefore 333 hours. Based on a 37.5 hour week, this is equivalent to 8.9 nurses. Allowing one nurse to cover the ward for twelve hours, seven days a week would require 84 hours of nursing time. If the total nursing time available (333 hours) is divided by that required for one nurse (84 hours), the formula allows four nurses to be on duty at any time during the day. In a 20-bedded ward this is equivalent to one nurse per five beds. On a similar calculation, the allowance for an acute (assessment) female geriatric ward of 20 similarly dependent patients would be 406 hours and this would allow (by similar calculations) one nurse per 4.2 beds. It is interesting that these figures are generally similar to the mean figures shown here (4.1 for beds per nurse for acute wards, and 4.6 for long-stay wards).

The second question—whether it is reasonable that there should be enormous variation in standards of nursing staff numbers between different types of wards—remains a subject for debate. The Scottish Home and Health Department in their 1969 report, assessed long-stay geriatric wards as requiring lower numbers of nurses than acute geriatric wards. Magid and Rhys Hearn[5], calculating the workload from their base line standard, used long-stay wards as the norm (100 per cent) and indicated that the direct workload in acute geriatric wards was 126 per cent, in psychogeriatric wards 90 per cent and in rehabilitation wards 75 per cent. However, they point out that in the case of rehabilitation wards their base line care policy (BLCP) makes no allowance for rehabilitative care—which is ironic to say the least. In fact, the nature of nursing in acute, rehabilitation and long-stay geriatric wards is so different that further studies are needed to validate or refute the principle that long-stay wards require fewer nurses than acute geriatric wards, and the position of rehabilitation wards needs to be determined.

As far as geographical variations are concerned, there can be no justification for such variation between different hospitals and different parts of the country, and yet this variation is between 200 per cent and 300 per cent between the best and the worst staffed wards.

The third question is whether student nurses should gain their geriatric experience (or at least some of it) on long-stay wards or not. We have shown (Table 42) that only 10 per cent of long-stay wards have student nurses compared to 33 per cent of AR wards and 27 per cent of acute wards. The figure for rehabilitation wards alone is 21 per cent. While any experience in geriatric wards must be good for student nurses (assuming the quality of care is good) it would seem likely that the most unique experience in geriatric nursing is to be obtained in rehabilitation and long-stay wards. The three functions of nursing acutely ill old people, nursing patients undergoing rehabilitation and nursing those requiring long-term care, are completely different and the various chapters in this book that deal with these activities indicate this. The management in acute wards is most akin to that in acute medical wards where the students already have a lot of exposure. Hill and Milnes[8] examined nursing hours in a series of geriatric wards and showed that the more immobile people there were on a ward, the fewer hours were worked by trained staff and learners—findings which are in line with ours reported here. It is concluded, therefore, that if learners are to spend only eight to ten weeks in geriatric wards most of this time should be involved with rehabilitation and long-stay patients.

7 Occupational therapy

Introduction

Since its earliest days geriatric medicine has been in partnership with occupational therapy. Geriatricians were among the first specialists to appreciate the scope and potential of occupational therapists and occupational therapists have contributed a great deal to the development of the specialty of geriatrics. In the 1950s and early 1960s the emphasis was on recreational therapy but as rehabilitation achieved greater prominence in the work of geriatric departments, the role of occupational therapists began to change. Now most occupational therapists would see their major function as the assessment of disability, teaching patients methods of overcoming their disabilities as they perform the ordinary activities of daily life, and altering the environment where necessary to assist the disabled person at home. These developments have been associated with changes in the structure of occupational therapy departments. Most departments now include a model bedroom, bathroom and kitchen and some, indeed, a flat where patients can demonstrate their ability (or inability) to live independently before they are actually discharged home. The occupational therapist's work involved going into the community to advise on alterations and adaptations to patients' homes as well as taking patients back to their homes in order to assess their functional capabilities in the home setting. All of this has marked a considerable development in the profession of occupational therapy and, in many cases, the more recreational aspects of the work have been diminished or lost altogether. This might be seen as something of an over-reaction and no doubt the swing will correct itself as time goes by.

The output of occupational therapists is fairly static in this country. At present there are 16 schools from which 736 occupational therapists qualify every year. The value of occupational therapy has now become apparent in almost all fields of medicine, particularly orthopaedics, general surgery, psychiatry and paediatrics. Throughout the last fifteen years there has also been an increase in employment of occupational therapists by social service departments. Because of this, the supply of occupational therapists no longer meets the demand and there has been a development of occupational therapy aides, who figure very prominently in some departments of geriatric medicine. They are, however, untrained other than having in-service training in the department in which they are working.

Within geriatric units, occupational therapy departments are often situated in day hospitals or in association with the geriatric rehabilitation wards. Some therapists have developed special interests in stroke rehabilitation and in orthopaedic geriatric rehabilitation and others are particularly involved in psychogeriatrics.

Staffing levels

There is no agreement as to what constitutes a satisfactory norm for the number of occupational therapists in geriatric units. Present suggested levels vary from 0.27 to 0.4 occupational therapists per 1000 population 65 years and over[1,2,3] with an equal number of therapy aides to work with the trained staff. Lack of a definitive norm makes it difficult to assess whether various units are adequately staffed.

In an attempt to assess staffing requirements the occupational therapists in the geriatric units in the UK were asked in the third study to provide information about the numbers and grades of staff in post, whether they regarded this number as adequate to provide a reasonable service and how therapists distributed their time. Two hundred and sixty-seven occupational therapy departments were contacted and the response rate was 76 per cent.

Thirty-seven units (18 per cent) felt that they had adequate staffing levels to provide a reasonable service for their area. There were some differences in staff structure between those departments which regarded their staff as adequate and those which saw it as inadequate. The former had a higher proportion of trained staff (95 per cent of the 37 adequately staffed units had 31 per cent or more of their staff trained compared with 74 per cent of the inadequately staffed units). The mean number of therapists was 5.49 in the former and 4.25 in the latter and the mean number of trained therapists 2.80 compared with 1.91. Another difference is that rather more of the adequately staffed units had a head occupational therapist (57 per cent compared with 46 per cent). However, only 48 per cent of all the geriatric units replying had a head occupational therapist and 34 per cent a senior I grade. Since there is likely to be some overlap in these units (some having both a head and a senior I) it seems that at least 20 per cent of departments have neither. Nearly every unit had a senior II grade occupational therapist in post. About half of the therapists were aides which fits in with the generally recommended distribution of staff, that is, one aide to

Occupational therapy

support each trained therapist. There was, of course, quite wide variation. Thus in 22 per cent of the units 70 per cent or more of the staff were untrained whereas in another 30 per cent of units more than 60 per cent of the staff were trained occupational therapists (Table 45).

Table 45 **Occupational therapy staffing levels in geriatric units and therapists' opinions of adequacy of provision**

	Therapists' opinions of staffing level					
	Adequate		*Inadequate*		*Total*	
	Units	Therapists	Units	Therapists	Units	Therapists
Number	37	203.2	166	706.2	203	909.4
Staff grade	%	%	%	%	%	%
Head	57	10	46	10	48	0
Senior I	32	7	34	7	34	7
Senior II	97	11	98	13	98	12
Basic	81	23	48	15	54	17
Aide	97	49	73	55	91	54
Trained staff		51		45		46
% Staff Trained	%		%		%	
<30%	5		26		22	
31–60%	59		45		48	
>60%	35		28		30	

How many occupational therapists are required?

How realistic was this assessment by occupational therapists of the adequacy of their staffing levels? It might be expected that asking any professional group whether they had sufficient staff would result in an over-estimation of requirements. In fact this did not appear to occur. Demographic information about the population served was available for 24 (63 per cent) of the occupational therapy departments responding to the questionnaire. This shows that the mean number of staff in those units with adequate staffing levels was significantly higher per elderly population than in those with inadequate levels (Table 46). However, the estimate of adequacy by staff of the units regarding themselves as inadequately staffed represented a higher overall level than pertained in the units regarding themselves as adequately staffed. This may have been either because the two groups have different needs or because in the presence of very low staffing levels the required need was over-estimated. Nevertheless even these levels were well below the present norms recommended by the British Medical Association (BMA) and the British Geriatrics Society (BGS). If the mean of

75

these two groups (those which are 'adequate' and the level estimated as adequate by those who presently regard their staff as inadequate) is taken the figures are as follows:

total occupational therapy staff—0.32 per 1000 population aged 65 plus;

trained occupational therapy staff—0.17 per 1000 population aged 65 plus (Table 47).

These levels are very much lower than those suggested by the BMA and the BGS[1,2] of 0.27–0.4 for trained and 0.55–0.72 for untrained staff.

Table 46 Required occupational therapist levels according to staff satisfaction with present staffing levels

	Present staffing levels							
	Sufficient			Insufficient				
		Present level			Required level			
	n	Mean	SEM	n	Mean	SEM	Mean	SEM
Trained OT/pop	24	0.15	0.02	103	0.09	0.01	0.18	0.01
Total OT/pop	24	0.31	0.03	103	0.21	0.01	0.32	0.02
Trained OT/bed	24	0.02	0.00	103	0.01	0.00	0.02	0.00
Total OT/bed	24	0.04	0.01	104	0.03	0.00	0.04	0.00

Table 47 Occupational therapist staffing levels in geriatric medicine—present and required

		Present level		Required level		Present norm*
	n	Mean	SEM	Mean	SEM	
Trained OT/pop	127	0.01	0.01	0.17	0.01	0.27–0.4
Total OT/pop	127	0.23	0.01	0.32	0.02	0.55–0.72
Trained OT/bed	128	0.01	0.00	0.02	0.00	0.027–0.04
Total OT/bed	128	0.03	0.00	0.04	0.00	0.055–0.072

*Norm = therapists/1000 population aged 65 and over

To consider the impact of these various suggested figures they may be compared to the numbers of occupational therapists at present in post in the areas from which returns were made. The total population aged 65 plus of those areas regarding themselves as adequately staffed was 791,000 and those regarding themselves as inadequately staffed was 3,250,000. The total number of occupational therapy staff in the former is 225 (and since this is regarded as adequate there is no shortfall). The total staff in the latter is 920 and compared with the staffing regarded as necessary to provide an adequate service in these areas, there is a shortfall of 305 (Table 48).

Occupational therapy

This consists of 244 trained therapists and 61 therapy aides. Since the population covered was about half that of the UK, for purposes of a rough estimate these figures can be doubled.

Table 48   Occupational therapists in geriatric medicine in the study area

	Occupational therapists numbers		
	Adequate	Inadequate	Total
Population	791.8	3250.3	4042.1
Beds	5818	26622	32440
Trained in post	106.8	266.8	373.6
Aides in post	118.6	348.3	466.9
'Adequate' levels			
Trained	106.8	510.6	617.3
Aides	118.6	409.8	528.4
Trained shortage	0	243.8	243.8
Aides shortage	0	61.5	61.5
Total shortage	0	305.3	305.3

Information on staffing levels is also available from the questionnaires completed by consultant geriatricians in the first study (Table 49). There are quite marked differences between the four countries of the UK. Three per cent of units had no occupational therapist and an additional 58 per cent had fewer than 0.1 occupational therapists per 1000 population 65 years and over. Northern Ireland in general had the highest provision of occupational therapists.

Based on a level of 0.17 occupational therapists per 1000 population over 65 years (see above), 84 per cent of units are deficient. If all units were to reach this level about 590 extra occupational therapists would be required. This compares with the shortfall estimated by occupational therapists themselves of about 610 (see above). However, this figure is equivalent to one sixth of all the available occupational therapists in the UK. Such levels would require additional schools of occupational therapy to be built since it is unlikely that expansion of present schools can achieve this level. It must also be recognised that there are shortages of therapists in other specialties. Any significant move to geriatric medicine by therapists working in other fields is thus highly improbable.

In view of the enormity of this estimated shortage, thought must be given to alternative methods of providing suitable services for the elderly. One suggestion is to train nurses in rehabilitation techniques to carry out the basic work and thus allow therapists to use their specialised skills. Such training might be incorporated in nurses' basic training, be part of the post-basic course in geriatric nursing or be a separate post-basic course. Another suggestion has

Table 49 Occupational therapists in geriatric units in the UK

	England	Wales	Scotland	N Ireland	UK
Trained OT/population					
No of units	145	13	26	8	192
Mean OT/pop	0.10	0.08	0.11	0.15	0.10
SEM	0.01	0.02	0.00	0.03	0.00
Range:	%	%	%	%	%
None	2	8	8	0	3
<0.1	60	61	53	38	58
−0.17	23	23	19	25	23
−0.25	11	0	12	25	11
>0.25	3	8	8	13	5
Known unfilled posts	109.7	13.2	6.5	2.0	131.4
Total (trained + aides) OT/pop					
No of units	143	13	24	8	188
Mean OT/pop	0.22	0.22	0.22	0.32	0.22
SEM	0.01	0.05	0.03	0.09	0.01
Shortage of trained OT from norm of:					
0.17 OT/pop					
Study area	392	29	36	3	
Projected total	504	38	41	4	
0.26 OT/pop					
Study area	882	58	94	15	
Projected total	1134	77	105	21	
0.4 OT/pop					
Study area	1644	103	184	35	
Projected total	2133	136	204	47	
Total trained OT (all specialties)	2718	142	348	151	

been the development of a generic therapist for the elderly who will use a combination of physiotherapy, occupational therapy and nursing skills. This concept was originally suggested by the World Health Organization to deal with all age groups but may be specially relevant for the elderly.

Style of practice and occupational therapy staffing

There seemed to be little difference between the styles of geriatric practice (Table 50) as to the number of therapists in post except that those working in mixed acute and rehabilitation with separate long-stay units (AR/L) had very low staffing levels. Since these were mainly in rural areas and small towns the low staffing levels might have been related to the difficulty in appointing staff rather than the influence of the style of practice. The levels proposed as necessary to provide an adequate service were much higher for trained staff in those units with separate rehabilitation wards. It may well be that the perception of occupational therapists working in units with separate rehabilitation wards is one in which their own role is emphasised and therefore they see the need for higher staffing levels. On the other hand, the designation of wards for rehabilitation may result in a greater number of patients being selected for intensive rehabilitation and a real increase in the workload.

Table 50 Style of geriatric unit and occupational therapist staffing levels

	Style			
	A/R/L	AR/L	A/RL	ARL
n	33	50	16	29
Trained OT/pop				
Present				
Mean	0.11	0.09	0.11	0.11
SEM	0.01	0.01	0.02	0.01
Required				
Mean	0.20	0.15	0.18	0.16
SEM	0.02	0.01	0.03	0.01
Total OT/pop				
Present				
Mean	0.24	0.21	0.24	0.25
SEM	0.02	0.02	0.03	0.02
Required				
Mean	0.36	0.29	0.32	0.31
SEM	0.03	0.03	0.04	0.03

Occupational staffing and workload

Comparing occupational therapy staffing with bed provision per 1000 population aged 65 plus, it is seen (Table 51) that units with adequate staffing levels had more occupational therapists when the bed levels were 7.5–10.5 per population than either above or below this figure. Since those units with more than 10.5 beds per 1000 population 65 years and over were more likely to have a higher proportion of long-stay beds, it is understandable that there is not a direct correlation between the number of therapists and the number of beds. By contrast, in those units where the therapists thought the staffing was inadequate, the levels they thought necessary were higher in those departments which did have more than 10.5 beds per 1000 population (and thus may be expected to have a larger proportion of long-term care patients). They certainly have a much lower discharge rate than units with lower bed ratios. This may indicate a greater desire of those working in the units regarded as insufficiently staffed to become further involved in long-term care wards. A larger number of therapists was also required when the turnover per bed (though not per population) was the lowest. In fact the more rapid the turnover of patients per bed the lower was the staffing level. It may be that where the interest is biased towards acute medical aspects of care, fewer therapists are required than when greater emphasis is placed on rehabilitation and the management of the chronically disabled old person. Similar patterns were found for the total (trained plus aides) therapists required (Table 51). It would therefore seem that the number of therapists thought to be required depends to some extent on the particular interests of the consultant geriatrician in charge of the unit and the style of practice.

How do occupational therapists spend their time?

The occupational therapists were asked to estimate the amount of time they spent in different types of activity (group therapy,

Table 51 Occupational therapist staffing levels related to geriatric unit characteristics

	Mean number of occupational therapists/population				
	Sufficient	Insufficient		Total	
	Present	Present	Required	Present	Required
Trained OT					
Beds/pop					
<7.5	0.11	0.09	0.18	0.09	0.16
−10.5	0.18	0.08	0.16	0.10	0.16
>10.5	0.15	0.11	0.21	0.11	0.21
Discharges/pop					
<35	0.14	0.09	0.19	0.11	0.18
−45	0.14	0.11	0.20	0.12	0.18
>45	0.18	0.07	0.16	0.09	0.16
Discharges/bed					
<3.5	0.17	0.11	0.21	0.12	0.20
−6	0.14	0.09	0.18	0.10	0.17
>6	0.14	0.07	0.15	0.09	0.14
Total OT (trained + aides)					
Beds/pop					
<7.5	0.29	0.19	0.30	0.21	0.30
−10.5	0.33	0.20	0.30	0.23	0.30
>10.5	0.24	0.27	0.40	0.26	0.38
Discharges/pop					
<35	0.28	0.22	0.34	0.23	0.33
−45	0.28	0.23	0.34	0.24	0.32
>45	0.41	0.17	0.28	0.21	0.30
Discharges/bed					
<3.5	0.31	0.25	0.38	0.26	0.37
−6	0.26	0.20	0.31	0.21	0.30
>6	0.37	0.17	0.26	0.21	0.29

individual therapy, case conferences or ward rounds, administration, travel and home visits). Although an estimate is not a reliable method of assessing the way the time is distributed it would have been impossible to carry out a detailed work audit in so many units. Such an audit would necessarily be for a short period only and might not allow for day-to-day fluctuation in the work pattern. Table 52 shows that about half of the trained occupational therapists' time is spent on individual patient treatment. Of the rest about 10 per cent is spent on group therapy, 10 per cent on case conferences and 9 per cent on home visits. This leaves about 11 per cent spent on administration and 5 per cent on travelling between wards and hospitals. Within these figures there were quite wide variations. About one third of departments did no group work at all and 3 per cent did no individual therapy. Attendance at case conferences varied between none (in 7 per cent of departments) and over 12 per cent of therapists' time (in 26 per cent of departments). Similarly, 37 per cent of units spent more than 12 per cent of occupational therapy time on administration. These non-patient contact activities, especially administration, may offer some potential for rationalisation of treatment time in some units.

Table 52   Proportion of time spent on different activities by trained occupational therapists

% time	Activity (% of units)					
	Group therapy	Indiv therapy	Case conf	Admin	Travel	Home visit
	%	%	%	%	%	%
0	35	3	7	5	26	14
− 4	7		10	7	20	10
− 8	16	1	24	22	30	18
− 12	12		30	26	11	28
− 16	8		13	16	5	9
− 20	5	3	8	16	2	6
− 40	8	22	5	5	1	4
− 60	4	48	0	0	0	2
>60	2	20	0	0	0	0
Unknown	2	2	2	3	4	8
Mean	9.7	49.2	10.1	11.4	5.0	9.1

There was also a very wide variation in the number of home visits. Fourteen per cent of units did not carry out home visits while 11 per cent spent more than 16 per cent of their time on this form of assessment (Table 52). In general 39 per cent of patients had pre-discharge assessment home visits and 15 per cent discharge home visits (Table 53). Here again there was a wide variation between the

Table 53 Discharge planning

	% of units	
% of patients	Assessment home visit	Discharge home visit
None	5	31
<10%	21	32
−30%	24	17
−50%	17	8
−70%	7	2
>70%	21	5
Not stated	4	4

Mean % of patients assessment home visit = 38.5; discharge home visit = 15.4.

units. About one quarter of units carried out assessment home visits on less than 10 per cent of their patients while about one fifth of units carried out these visits on over 70 per cent of their patients. Discharge home visits, that is, assessments of home circumstances made at the time of discharge, were less frequently carried out, though in 11 per cent of units this was done for over 50 per cent of the patients.

The therapists were also asked to estimate the amount of treatment time they spent on different activities. Table 54 shows that the greatest amount of time was spent on assessment (26 per cent) and on training in the activities of daily living (28 per cent). Very little time was spent on testing and treating perceptual disorders or on diversional activities. Once again there was wide variation between the units. For instance, about one third of units spent less than 10 per cent of treatment time on assessment while a

Table 54 Proportion of treatment time spent on different activities by trained occupational therapists

			Activity			
% Time	Assess	ADL	Perceptual training	Aids provision and assessment	Diversional activity	Remedial therapy
	%	%	%	%	%	%
None	5	3	23	5	50	28
−10	11	9	61	43	33	25
−20	26	14	3	24	4	12
−30	20	28	1	11	3	5
−50	18	26	0	4	2	2
>50	7	3	0	2	0	0
Unknown	12	12	12	12	10	9
Mean*	25.8	28.4	4.7	14.5	4.5	7.7

*Mean of the known values

Occupational therapy

similar proportion spent more than 40 per cent of time doing so. Half the units denied carrying out diversional activities though a few did seem to spend a large proportion of their time this way. This may be because occupational therapists have had to make an effort to be seen to have skills other than basket-making and filling in the patients' time. On the other hand it may simply indicate the varying perceptions of different therapists as to their priorities.

What would occupational therapists do if they had more staff?

In view of the marked shortage of therapists it is useful to know what work would be carried out if there were an increase in the number of staff.

The therapists were asked what activities or services they would like to improve if they had more staff. Table 55 shows the results. Replies to this question were received from all but two of the 'inadequately' staffed units but only 65 per cent of those with adequate levels. There were slight differences in emphasis between the two groups. Those with adequate staffing levels would generally increase the amount of treatment given to individual patients, increase the work on long-stay wards and carry out more home visits. Those with inadequate staffing levels listed treating more long-stay patients and giving more group therapy as their main priorities, followed by increasing the amount of treatment, more home visits and more ADL treatment. In fact emphasis on more work among long-stay patients tops the list in both groups.

In general, an increase in staff would probably not increase the amount of research or teaching carried out by occupational therapy departments. It would therefore seem that these activities would have to be carried out in a small number of specialist units.

The provision of aids

The therapists were asked who provided specific aids to daily living and what was the average time to obtain them. It can be seen from Table 56 that aids provided by the hospital were supplied much more quickly than those provided by social services. In some areas aids may take several months to be delivered—a highly unsatisfactory situation. Hospitals (although often supplied by social service departments in the first place) were more likely to provide simple aids such as special cutlery, plates and dressing aids. District nurses were more likely to provide commodes. Social services provided most toilet aids and chemical toilets although the latter were unavailable to 19 per cent of departments.

There is such wide variation in the time taken to obtain aids

Table 55 Areas of increased activity if more occupational therapists were available

	Therapists' opinion of staffing levels		
	Sufficient OT	Insufficient OT	Total
No of departments	37	166	203
Information available	24 (65%)	163 (98%)	16 (92%)
	%	%	%
General			
Treat more patients	0	13	11
Earlier treatment	0	1	1
Increase amount of treatment	8	27	23
Better assessment	4	9	7
More individual therapy	21	16	15
More group therapy	8	29	25
More ADL therapy	17	20	18
Maintenance therapy	0	2	1
Specialist therapy			
Stroke	4	4	3
Perceptual training	0	6	4
Reality orientation	17	12	11
Remedial activities	4	9	7
Recreational/social	4	10	8
Specific areas			
Day hospital	0	16	13
Domiciliary treatment	8	4	4
Residential homes	0	1	1
Home visits	17	27	24
Long-stay wards	21	31	27
Other activities			
Inter/intra departmental communication	4	1	1
Attend ward rounds	0	1	1
Counselling	0	5	4
In service training	4	3	3
Research	0	3	2

provided by social services that it is clear that not all local authorities are responding to the needs of the disabled in this regard. Part of this may be due to confusion and lack of communication but in many cases it is probably due to inadequate funding and poor coordination of services.

Discussion

The number of occupational therapists in geriatric units falls so far short of the levels recommended by the BMA and BGS that these must be regarded as totally unrealistic. A norm of 0.17 trained occupational therapists per 1000 population aged 65 years and over emerges as the occupational therapists' view of the numbers

Occupational therapy

required and is a somewhat more realistic goal. However over the next quarter century the demand will increase because of the growth of the population aged 75 and over and particularly of those aged 85 and over. Other solutions must therefore be sought which require careful research into the way in which occupational therapists work. Their work in long-stay wards, for instance, might with advantage be transferred to activities organisers (see page 49). Perhaps the same might apply to group therapy. These are solutions for occupational therapists to consider.

If aids are needed to enable disabled patients to return to their homes, any delay in their provision delays the patient's discharge from hospital. This is both regrettable for the patient and costly for the NHS. Where the hospital has a store of aids (usually provided by the social services department) the provision of the aid was quick. However, in some areas patients waited several months for even the simplest of aids to be provided by social services departments.

Table 56 Provision of aids

Aid	Hospital		Soc serv		Hospital + soc serv		District nurse		Not available
	%	Weeks	%	Weeks	%	Weeks	%	Weeks	%
Cutlery	54	0–1	19	1–32	25	1–16	—	—	—
Plates	55	0–2	20	1–32	23	1–16	—	—	—
Kitchen aids	33	0–2	35	1–32	28	1–52	—	—	1
Dressing aid	54	0–1	24	1–52	20	1–8	—	—	—
Bath aid	14	0–2	64	1–52	16	1–52	—	—	—
Toilet aid	13	1–4	53	1–32	19	1–16	11	1–4	—
Chairs	5	1–32	75	1–52	5	1–8	4	1–8	7
Commodes	2	0–1	20	1–16	1	0–1	51	1–16	2
Chem toilets	3	1–8	55	1–52	1	0–1	19	1–16	19
Ramps	2	4–8	97	1–52	2	1–32	—	—	—
Rails	4	1–32	96	1–52	2	1–32	—	—	—

8 Physiotherapy

Introduction

Physiotherapy is an important part of the total management of patients in geriatric units. The physiotherapists' major input is in relation to the rehabilitation of frail and disabled old people, both when they are inpatients and also in the day hospital. This involves work with stroke patients, those with fracture of the femur, osteoarthritis, amputation of a leg and Parkinsonism. Much of the work, however, will be elderly people who are unable to walk because of the effect of systemic disease, very often against a background of multiple pathology and general frailty. In addition to active rehabilitation, physiotherapists are involved in maintaining the level of independence which has been reached. This is often carried out in the day hospital, though in some cases it may be achieved by domiciliary physiotherapy.

The role of physiotherapy among long-stay patients is to maintain what ability they have and to advise according to changing needs for wheelchairs and appliances. There is thus a good deal of variation in the work of physiotherapists in geriatric departments, depending on the style of practice of the unit concerned and the extent to which the interdisciplinary team concept has been developed. In the face of such variation some difficulty is to be expected in assessing required staffing levels and describing the range of specific activities and equipment used by different departments.

In an attempt to define the present state of physiotherapy in geriatric medicine, as part of the fourth study, a postal questionnaire was sent to the senior physiotherapist of all the geriatric units in the UK. Replies were received from 73 per cent of the 268 units contacted. Information from this questionnaire, together with details from the other studies, has been used to build up a picture of the pattern of physiotherapy in geriatric units.

Since there is no agreement as to what constitutes a satisfactory staffing level for physiotherapy departments in geriatric units, it is difficult to discuss the adequacy of provision throughout the country. Norms suggested by various authorities such as the British Medical Association and the British Geriatrics Society[1,2,3] vary from 0.26 to 0.5 trained physiotherapists per 1000 population 65 years and over, supported by an equal number of physiotherapy aides.

To try to evaluate the number of physiotherapists required the therapists were asked in the fourth study: 'Do you feel that the staff you have is adequate to provide a reasonable service?', and, 'If not, how many additional staff would you require to provide a reasonable service?'

We recognise that these questions are open to wide interpretation but it is difficult to see how they could be more specific. There is no recognised workload for physiotherapy departments and much will depend on the specific needs of the individual area and the particular interests of the consultant in charge of the unit. Even a detailed work study in a small number of units would not represent the whole country when there is such wide variation in clinical practice, and would only cover a short period of time in a fluctuating work pattern. There is therefore some attraction in depending on the therapists' perceptions as long as the limitations are recognised.

Staffing levels

One hundred and ninety six departments completed the questionnaire. Of these, 81 regarded staffing levels as adequate, 115 as inadequate. Table 57 shows comparative staffing levels for these two groups. There is a difference in the number of therapists, both trained and untrained, per 1000 population 65 years and over. The average for all units is 0.25 therapists per 1000 population 65 years and over, of which 0.15 are trained. Table 57 also shows the different grades of staff in the two groups and indicates that there is little difference in the proportion of staff in the different grades or in the percentage of the total staff who are trained. In fact, of course, those with adequate levels had about 22 per cent more trained staff than those with inadequate levels for the population to be covered.

How many physiotherapists are required?

Using the information from the therapists about their staffing numbers, those with adequate levels had, on average, 0.17 physiotherapists per 1000 population 65 years and over (Table 58) compared to 0.14 for those with inadequate staffing levels. When asked how many therapists would be required 'to provide a reasonable service' those with inadequate levels indicated that they would require numbers equivalent to 0.2 therapists per 1000 population 65 years and over. This was higher than the level of those units which felt that they had adequate staffing levels. This may be due to a real difference in the workload between the two groups or may indicate an over-estimation of the numbers required caused by the pressure of coping with so few staff.

British Geriatric Medicine in the 1980s

Table 57 Physiotherapy staffing on geriatric units related to therapists' opinions of adequacy of staffing levels

	Therapists' opinions of staffing level					
	Adequate		Inadequate		Total	
	Units	Therapists	Units	Therapists	Units	Therapists
Number	81	457.8	115	513.1	196	970.9
Staff grade	%	%	%	%	%	%
Suprin	44	7	43	10	44	9
Senior I	54	11	45	13	49	59
Senior II	79	19	64	19	70	19
Basic	80	25	66	21	72	23
Aides	94	38	81	38	86	38
Trained	96	62	100	62	98	62
% Trained						
<30%		1		4		3
−60%		42		39		45
>60%		57		57		57
Staff required						
Trained		0		192.7		192.7
Aides		0		43.1		43.1
Total		0		235.8		235.8
PT/pop						
Trained		0.171		0.140		0.151
Total		0.288		0.229		0.251

Table 58 Physiotherapist levels according to staff satisfaction with present staffing levels

	Present staffing levels				
	Sufficient		Insufficient		
			Present level		Required level
	n	Mean	n	Mean	Mean
Trained PT/pop	49	0.17	84	0.14	0.21
Total PT/pop	49	0.29	84	0.23	0.32
Trained PT/bed	50	0.02	85	0.02	0.03
Total PT/bed	50	0.03	85	0.03	0.04

Where there were inadequate staffing levels the therapists required 61 per cent more trained staff and 22 per cent more physiotherapy aides to reach levels which they would regard as adequate to provide a reasonable service.

If the figures for all the physiotherapists are combined (Table 59), the number of trained therapists was only 0.15 per population, compared to the norms suggested by the British Medical Associ-

Physiotherapy

Table 59 Physiotherapist staffing levels in geriatric medicine—present and required

	Present level		Required level	Present norm*
	n	Mean	Mean	Range
Trained PT/pop	133	0.15	0.19	0.26–0.5
Total PT/pop	133	0.25	0.31	0.35–0.7
Trained PT/bed	135	0.02	0.02	0.03–0.05
Total PT/bed	135	0.03	0.04	0.04–0.07

*Norm = therapists/1000 population aged 65 and over as suggested by BMA and BGS (see text)

Table 60 Physiotherapists in geriatric medicine in the study area

	Sufficient	Insufficient	Total
Population	1543	2627	4170
Beds	13088	23132	36220
Trained in post	263.51	354.08	617.59
Aides in post	168.55	230.13	398.68
'Adequate' levels			
Trained	263.51	516.31	779.82
Aides	168.55	265.83	434.38
Trained shortage	0	162.23	162.23
Total shortage	0	197.93	197.93

ation and British Geriatrics Society of 0.26 to .50 per population. However, if we take the levels the therapists would, on average, regard as being adequate to provide a reasonable service, then a norm of 0.19 trained physiotherapists per population is required, although there is a very wide range around this mean.

Table 60 puts numbers to these normative levels. It will be seen that for the population covered in the fourth study, 162.2 (21 per cent) more trained physiotherapists and 35.7 (9 per cent) more physiotherapy aides would be required to provide a service regarded by physiotherapists as adequate. Since the population covered is only about half that in the whole of the UK these figures can probably be doubled for national requirements.

Further evidence of this can be seen from our first study (Table 61). This shows the staffing ratios of physiotherapists as reported by the geriatricians for the four countries of the UK. Scotland and Northern Ireland had a higher provision of physiotherapists for the elderly population with England having the lowest provision. Overall, 89 per cent of units fell below 0.25, and 76 per cent below 0.19, physiotherapists per 1000 population 65 years and over. This was not compensated for by an increase in physiotherapy aides.

Table 61 Physiotherapy staff in geriatric units throughout the UK

	England	Wales	Scotland	N Ireland	UK
Trained PT/pop					
No of units	147	13	26	8	194
Mean PT/pop	0.140	0.153	0.166	0.163	0.146
Range:					
<0.15	64%	54%	54%	63%	62%
−0.19	14%	23%	8%	13%	14%
−0.25	13%	8%	19%	0	13%
>0.25	9%	15%	19%	25%	11%
Known unfilled posts	46.3	6.9	3.7	8.8	65.7
Total PT (trained + aides)/pop					
No of units	144	13	26	8	194
Mean/pop	0.24	0.27	0.23	0.35	0.24
Shortage of trained PT from norm of:					
0.19 PT/pop					
Study area	272	12	15	4	
Projected total	352	16	17	5	
0.25 PT/pop					
Study area	599	31	54	12	
Projected total	770	41	60	16	
0.5 PT/pop					
Study area	1960	112	214	46	
Projected total	2519	147	237	63	
Total trained PT (all specialties)	6832	356	983	264	

England, for instance, only had an average of 0.24 total (trained plus aides) therapists per 1000 population 65 years and over—about the level recommended for trained staff alone.

If the figures are projected to the total population in the UK, even using the therapists' suggested level of 0.19, about 390 additional trained therapists are required. This is about 5 per cent of the physiotherapists available for all specialties. In addition, within the reporting departments, there were 66 physiotherapy posts unfilled though funded, mostly in England. It is improbable that a shift in staff from other specialties would be possible since they are also regarded as understaffed.

To achieve a satisfactory number of therapists, according to these calculations, an expansion of present physiotherapy schools or, more likely, the development of new schools will be necessary. Alternative approaches would be to encourage trained therapists who are no longer working to return to practice either part-time or on a flexible time basis, or to train other disciplines, such as nurses, in the basic principles of rehabilitation thus allowing the therapists to concentrate their skills on the more specialist forms of therapy.

To return to the evidence from the fourth study relating to

Physiotherapy

adequacy of staffing levels, a pattern also emerged when comparing departments with different styles of geriatric practice (Table 62). Units with separate acute wards tended to have, and apparently require, more physiotherapists than those which combine acute and rehabilitation patients. The former includes both units with separate rehabilitation wards and those where rehabilitation and long-stay wards are combined. There is, however, wide variation within each group. Physiotherapists' views of the numbers required are likely to be influenced by their present staffing levels, although there may be a variation in the actual needs of different units reflecting, in turn, the bias of the geriatrician concerned.

Table 62 Style of geriatric unit and physiotherapist staffing levels

	Style			
	A/R/L	AR/L	A/RL	ARL
n	38	47	13	32
Trained PT/pop				
Present mean	0.16	0.14	0.17	0.15
Required mean	0.21	0.19	0.21	0.19
Total PT/pop				
Present mean	0.28	0.24	0.30	0.27
Required mean	0.34	0.31	0.34	0.31

The number of therapists per population does not directly relate to the therapists' workload since much will depend on the number of beds. However, the evidence from study three (Tables 58 and 59) suggests that those units dissatisfied with their staffing levels had fewer therapists per bed as well as per population.

Staffing levels increase quite strikingly with the number of beds per population (Table 63) as do the therapists' views of optimal levels. On the other hand there does not seem to be any direct pattern in relation to the number of discharges, either per population or per bed. This may be because a rapid turnover implies greater emphasis on the acute medical aspects of care while a low to moderate discharge rate implies an emphasis on longer-term care which may not require so much physiotherapy involvement.

One further influence on the number of therapists available may be the type of area in which the hospital is situated. In our first study we classified districts as cities, large towns, small towns, rural areas, 'retirement' areas and academic units. It appeared that the highest provision was in the cities, large towns and academic units with the lowest in small towns and 'retirement' areas. Perhaps therapists are more easily recruited in the larger urban areas, possibly because of employment opportunities for all members of the family. There

Table 63 Physiotherapy staffing levels related to geriatric unit characteristics

	Mean number of physiotherapists/population				
	Sufficient	Insufficient		Total	
	present	present	required	present	required
Trained					
Beds/pop					
<7.5	0.15	0.13	0.18	0.14	0.17
−10.5	0.17	0.14	0.20	0.15	0.19
>10.5	0.22	0.16	0.23	0.18	0.22
Discharges/pop					
<35	0.17	0.13	0.20	0.14	0.19
−45	0.19	0.15	0.22	0.17	0.20
>45	0.16	0.15	0.22	0.15	0.20
Discharges/bed					
<3.5	0.20	0.14	0.22	0.16	0.21
−6	0.16	0.15	0.20	0.15	0.19
>6	0.16	0.14	0.20	0.15	0.18
Total (trained + aides)					
Beds/pop					
<7.5	0.23	0.22	0.29	0.23	0.26
−10.5	0.30	0.23	0.31	0.26	0.31
>10.5	0.37	0.23	0.35	0.27	0.35
Discharges/pop					
<35	0.32	0.20	0.29	0.24	0.30
−45	0.28	0.22	0.29	0.25	0.29
>45	0.24	0.26	0.36	0.26	0.32
Discharges/bed					
<3.5	0.37	0.19	0.30	0.26	0.32
−6	0.26	0.23	0.31	0.24	0.30
>6	0.23	0.26	0.33	0.25	0.29

was, however, no corresponding diminution in the number of therapy aides; indeed, there was also a greater number of these per population in the cities than in the other types of area.

How do physiotherapists spend their time?

It is not easy to define the workload of physiotherapists in the NHS. They depend on referral of patients by doctors, whose perceptions of the role of physiotherapists vary considerably. As well, there has been very little research to define the role of physiotherapy in conditions which affect the elderly. What clinical research there is has usually been carried out on younger people. There are also considerable differences in physiotherapists' own perceptions of what is required. This is seen, for instance, in the wide variation in approaches to stroke rehabilitation. Some methods require intensive and long-term individual therapist-patient contact while others

Physiotherapy

concentrate on a rapid functional approach using aids and appliances.

It is therefore difficult to know whether staffing levels are appropriate. To gain some insight into the work pattern of physiotherapists on geriatric units the physiotherapists were asked to estimate the proportion of trained therapy time spent on the following activities: individual therapy, group therapy, ward rounds or case conferences, administration, record-keeping and travel. These results are shown in Table 64. About two thirds of physiotherapy time seems to be spent on individual patient therapy—90 per cent of units were spending at least 50 per cent of their time in this way. Group therapy occupied less than 10 per cent of therapist

Table 64   Proportion of time spent on different activities by trained physiotherapists

% time	Group therapy	Individual therapy	Ward round	Administration	Travel
	%	%	%	%	%
0	36	2	3	4	30
−10	29	0	39	59	56
−20	25	2	50	25	14
−30	5	2	7	1	0
−60	4	20	<1	0	<1
>60	<1	74	0	0	0
Mean	8.6%	67.9%	11.5%	8.8%	5.2%

time in the main and was not used at all in over one third of departments. On average, 11.5 per cent of therapist time was spent on ward rounds and case conferences, though in as many as one fifth of units therapists spent more than 15 per cent of their time on this activity. Important though communication and goal planning is, it must be questioned whether some of this time would not have been more profitably spent on patient contact. Similarly, 9 per cent of time was spent on administration with as many as 36 per cent of units spending more than 10 per cent of all trained therapist time on record-keeping and administration. A clerk or secretary to the therapy department (possibly shared with other therapy departments) might release therapists for more direct patient therapy.

About 5 per cent of therapist time was spent travelling between wards and hospitals. A slight increase in staffing levels may decrease the need for so many areas to be covered by individual therapists, thereby reducing travelling time and allowing scarce resources to be deployed much more efficiently. The beneficial effect might well be disproportionately greater than the cost.

What would physiotherapists do if they had more staff?

On the assumption that therapists were limited in what they could achieve because of low staffing levels the physiotherapists were asked 'If you had more staff what additional activities or service would you like to be able to provide?' Table 65 shows the different opinions expressed by those who felt that they had an adequate number of staff and those who felt they did not. Only 54 per cent of those with adequate staffing levels replied to the question compared to 94 per cent of those with inadequate staffing levels.

The greatest emphasis for those with adequate staffing levels would be to increase the amount of domiciliary treatment sessions (48 per cent of units). Treatment of long-stay patients comes second (32 per cent), followed by the development of specialist stroke techniques (27 per cent), of group therapy (23 per cent) and of home assessment visits (20 per cent).

Table 65 Areas of increased activity if more physiotherapists were available

	Therapists' opinion of staffing levels		
	Adequate	*Inadequate*	*Total*
No of departments	81	115	196
Information available	44 (54%)	108 (94%)	152 (78%)
	%	%	%
General			
Better assessment	2	5	4
Earlier treatment	2	1	1
Increased intensity therapy	18	48	39
Increase individual therapy	5	14	11
Increase group therapy	23	34	31
Treat more patients	0	4	3
More follow-up	0	3	2
More outpatient therapy	2	16	12
More maintenance therapy	2	3	3
Specialist therapy			
Stroke	27	16	19
Psychogeriatrics	0	4	3
Specific areas			
Domiciliary treatment	48	17	26
Residential homes	14	6	9
Home visits	20	21	21
Long-stay wards	32	28	30
Other activities			
Inter/intradepartmental communication	2	4	3
Relative support groups	2	6	5
Attend ward rounds	0	4	3
In-service training	7	11	10
Research	2	3	3

Physiotherapy

A different order of priorities was expressed by those units with insufficient staffing levels. Increasing the intensity of treatment (48 per cent of units) and the amount of group activities (34 per cent) were cited most frequently, followed by increased activity on long-stay wards (28 per cent), home assessment visits (21 per cent), domiciliary treatment (17 per cent) and outpatient therapy (16 per cent).

Very few departments said they would treat more patients (4 per cent) or start treatment earlier (1 per cent). It therefore seems that an increase in staff would increase the quality of treatment rather than the number of patients treated, probably because the number of patients being treated is limited by the number of beds rather than the total population in need. Although most patients received treatment this does not imply that they received adequate amounts of therapy. Almost certainly the amount of treatment is more important than the simple provision of therapy. This has been shown to be the case for stroke rehabilitation.[4]

It is also notable that only 3 per cent of all departments would become involved in research. This is important since few physiotherapy techniques have been validated. One hope for the future is that better assessment of the techniques and equipment used in physiotherapy will result in greater efficiency and effectiveness. Our findings suggest that research posts will have to be separately funded in specialist centres if the work of therapists is to be evaluated.

It is noteworthy that an area not usually regarded as attractive to therapists—long-stay care—was so frequently cited as a priority. The reason for this is not clear, but may arise from the feeling that some patients require long-stay care because of inadequate amounts of therapy. This suggests that increasing the amount of therapy given to these 'slow stream' patients might result in a greater number of discharges. If so, this would be an important contribution as the pressure on geriatric beds increases over the next 20 years. Many therapists also believe—and there is plenty of clinical experience to support their view—that increased physical activity improves the quality of life for long-stay patients. More physiotherapy on long-stay wards would therefore have an effect not necessarily measurable by increased bed turnover.

Equipment available to physiotherapy departments

Physiotherapy consists mainly of individual therapist-patient contact. There is, however, a large amount of equipment available to physiotherapists. Table 66 shows the equipment which was available to the departments which replied to the questionnaire.

Table 66 Physiotherapy equipment used in geriatric units

Equipment	%
Infrared irradiation	91
Ice	82
Ultraviolet	70
Wax baths	63
Ultrasound	62
Short-wave diathermy	42
TENS	22
'Ozone'	19
Interferential therapy	10
Hydrocollator	9
Faradism	3
Hydrotherapy	1
Electromagnetic induction coil	1
Inflatable splints	79
Exercise bicycle	67
Intermittent pneumatic compression	64
Post amputation mobility aid	60
Standing frames	52
Suspension frame	10
Treadmill	6
Vibrator	3
Walking harness	1
Shoulder wheel	1

Most units used infrared irradiation, ice therapy, inflatable splints and ultraviolet therapy. About two thirds of the departments had wax baths, ultrasound therapy, exercise bicycles and intermittent pneumatic compression therapy. The post-amputation mobility aid (PAM) was available in 60 per cent of units and standing frames in about half. Other equipment, such as short-wave diathermy, transcutaneous electric stimulation and interferential therapy, was available in less than half the units while only one unit had a hydrotherapy pool. This may be because therapists regard direct patient contact as most important or because physiotherapy departments in geriatric units are not being provided with important equipment for their work. There is unfortunately very little evidence derived from research to show which equipment is essential or even of value.

Therapists also have differing views on simple devices such as walking aids (Table 67). Walking sticks are used by nearly all departments but quadsticks or tripods are less popular. Elbow, axilla and gutter crutches are rarely used for the elderly. The frame is almost universally used but the triangular frame, although probably easier to manipulate in the home, is less often used. Wheeled and forearm resting frames are also relatively unpopular. Usage varies widely for each aid. For instance, a tripod is frequently

Physiotherapy

used by 23 per cent of units and never used in 16 per cent; wheeled frames are used frequently by 38 per cent and never by 5 per cent of units. There seems to be a lack of consensus as to what is the most appropriate form of aid. This again suggests the need for further rehabilitation research.

Pressure sore therapy

Although the treatment of pressure sores is often considered a nursing procedure there are a number of physiotherapy techniques which are thought to improve healing. Table 68 shows the techniques which were used by the departments in this study.

Ultraviolet light was the most frequent form of treatment, though used by only 29 per cent of departments. The next most popular forms of treatment were ultrasound, 'ozone' therapy and ice. The evidence for the effectiveness of most of these techniques is, as yet, lacking.

Table 67 Frequency of use of walking aids in geriatric rehabilitation

	Frequency of use				
	Frequently	Occa-sionally	Rarely	Never	Not stated
Aid	%	%	%	%	%
Stick	76	23	2	0	0
Quadstick	30	33	25	10	1
Tripod	23	33	28	16	<1
Elbow crutches	2	21	57	21	<1
Gutter crutches	<1	19	55	25	<1
Axilla crutches	0	3	26	72	<1
Frame	99	0	0	<1	0
Triangular frame	7	24	30	37	2
Wheeled frame	38	44	12	5	1
Forearm resting frame	21	60	16	3	0

Table 68 Equipment used in treating pressure sores

	%
Ultraviolet light	28.6
Ultrasound	16.3
'Ozone'	12.8
Ice	10.7
Infrared	6.1
Oxygen	3.6
Air	3.1
Short wave diathermy	1.5
Connective tissue massage	0.5

Stroke rehabilitation

There has probably been more written about techniques of stroke rehabilitation than any other condition. The development of neurophysiological approaches to stroke rehabilitation has produced enthusiasts in stroke management. By far the most popular approach is that of the Bobath concept (Table 69) with almost every geriatric unit in the UK using some of these ideas in the rehabilitation of the stroke patient. Most units also utilised parts of other concepts. Proprioceptive neuromuscular facilitation (PNF) was the next most popular, perhaps surprisingly, since even many PNF advocates would regard this technique as having little to offer stroke patients. The other popular approach was that described by Margaret Johnstone which uses a combination of neurophysiological positioning techniques and some specialist equipment.

Table 69 Rehabilitation techniques used in stroke therapy

	%
Bobath	97.5
PNF	67.4
Johnstone	57.7
Rood	21.9
Brunnstrom	5.1
Conductive education	1.0
Peto	1.0
Frenkel	0.5

The difference between these techniques or approaches is largely one of emphasis. The Bobath approach emphasises the inhibition of abnormal reflex patterns; the Brunnstrom approach (popular on the European continent) uses the abnormal reflexes and automatic responses to encourage recovery of motor patterns; the Rood approach (more popular in the USA) encourages the use of stimuli to produce normal reactions; and proprioceptive neuromuscular facilitation uses the positioning of joints to facilitate voluntary mass muscle contraction. They all have in common an emphasis on neurophysiological sequencing of human motor development and attempts to modify motor activity by inhibition or facilitation of reflex activity. They all stress the importance of sensation, use repetition, encourage activity of the affected side using a bilateral approach and have a high level of therapist-patient contact time.

It seems obvious that few departments were purely orientated towards one specific technique and most used a mixture of approaches according to needs. This is not to say that some units did not have certain therapists who specialised in one particular concept, for example the Bobath approach.

Physiotherapy

Although stroke rehabilitation is generally thought of as being intensely therapist-patient contact orientated, there is a large amount of equipment which has a potential use. Table 70 shows the type of equipment used by different units. Frames and walking sticks were the most popular. It is of interest that, although stroke therapy textbooks decry the use of a walking stick because of its tendency to encourage poor walking patterns, most units did in fact use them although 42 per cent compromised by using a long stick or pole for balance rather than weight bearing. It is similarly of interest that quadsticks were so popular in spite of the present teaching against their use.

The inflatable splint was popular (75 per cent) and there seems to be interest (45 per cent of departments) in the use of pneumatic intermittent compression in the treatment of stroke.

Calipers are still used in two thirds of departments for leg splinting and have not been as fully replaced by the lighter splints as is generally thought.

Table 70   Equipment used in stroke rehabilitation

	%
Inflatable splints	75.0
Slings	69.9
Caliper	64.3
Ankle splints	46.4
Other splints	38.3
Swedish knee cage	10.2
Pneumatic intermittent compression	45.4
Ice	1.5
Vibration	1.5
Walking stick:	
normal length	82.7
long length/pole	41.8
Frame	82.1
Quadstick	76.5
Wheeled frame	58.7
Gutter frame	49.0
Pulpit frame	38.8
Single-handed frame	8.2
Arjo walker	2.0

Slings to prevent drag on the unprotected shoulder joint in stroke patients have both advocates and critics. As many as 70 per cent of units used slings. As can be seen from Table 71, the old-fashioned triangular bandage is rarely used. The two most popular types of sling are the figure of eight and the collar and cuff; the former is generally regarded as the most satisfactory by stroke specialists.

There is now considerable literature on the rehabilitation of the stroke patient, yet some approaches generally regarded as obsolete,

Table 71 Slings used for arm support in hemiplegia

	%
Slings not used	30.1
Figure of eight	24.5
Collar and cuff	21.9
Axilla roll	2.6
Triangular bandage	3.6
Other named—various	6.1
Type not stated	13.8

Table 72 Distances between geriatric units and limb-fitting centres

Miles	%
−10	21.9
−25	44.4
−40	21.4
>40	12.8
Not stated	2.0

Table 73 Assessment for wheelchair provision

Physiotherapist	27.0
Occupational therapist	41.3
PT/OT	29.6
ALAC	3.1

such as certain slings, calipers and quadsticks, are still being used. This may indicate a realistic approach to certain difficult situations which do not respond to textbook techniques, or it may indicate the necessity for continuing education to allow therapists to keep abreast of current developments.

Wheelchairs and limb-fitting centres

Wheelchairs are provided by artificial limb and appliance centres (ALAC), which may be many miles away from the district hospital (Table 72). About one third of the departments in the study were more than 25 miles from their nearest ALAC. Probably because of this, most units seemed to have arrangements at their local hospital for assessment of patients for wheelchairs. Although the application form for a wheelchair has to be signed by a doctor, it appears that the doctor was involved in the actual assessment in very few units. In 41 per cent of units (Table 73) the occupational therapist assessed the patient for a wheelchair and in 30 per cent of cases the assessment was made jointly by physiotherapists and occupational therapists.

Discussion

Only about one third of the physiotherapy departments believed that they had sufficient staff to provide a reasonable service. Even so the staffing levels they felt they required were, in general, below the levels recommended previously by the British Geriatrics Society and the British Medical Association. To achieve the levels recommended by these organisations, between 890 and 3000 additional therapists would be required—an increase of 11 per cent to 36 per cent over current levels. No matter how desirable these norms are they are obviously unachievable. Even to achieve the level of 0.19 trained therapists which the physiotherapists regard as reasonable (not ideal) would require about 390 more trained physiotherapists. This could only be achieved by expanding present physiotherapy schools or opening new ones. These figures are only analysed in relation to geriatric medicine but the available evidence seems to be that other specialties are equally understaffed. Some move toward this goal is required urgently. Other approaches should also be sought. Therapists who ceased practice when they left work to have children and who have not returned as their children have grown older form one potential group for increasing the pool of working therapists. A recruitment campaign and special courses for reorientation are required.

Another approach is to train nurses in basic rehabilitation techniques. This has two advantages. The first is that if the basic techniques of rehabilitation were routinely practised by nurses then trained therapists could be released for more specialist work. The second advantage is that rehabilitation cannot be regarded as an activity that happens only in the physiotherapy or occupational therapy departments but is a 24-hour process. It is therefore essential that nurses continue the same techniques used by the therapists if the patient is to avoid being confused by conflicting advice. Therapists are likely to feel threatened by such a suggestion but those working in well-organised multidisciplinary teams have long recognised the benefit of a team approach to rehabilitation. It would probably be appropriate to have a post-basic qualification of rehabilitation nursing for a relatively small number of nurses, especially those in charge of wards which have a high rehabilitation content. Patients would benefit from the consistent team approach, nurses would gain a greater satisfaction from their rehabilitation work and therapists would be able to concentrate their specialist expertise to the advantage of the patient.

Most of the departments in the study units seemed to have the basic physiotherapy equipment though there was a wide variation in access to other than basic appliances. This may indicate that physiotherapy for the elderly is largely a patient contact therapy. It may also imply the low provision of 'tools for the job' or reflect the variety of opinions held by physiotherapists concerning the value of specialist equipment. This can be seen, for instance, in the different approaches to the use of equipment in stroke rehabilitation. Some of the equipment and aids used, for example slings or calipers in stroke, raise the question as to whether there is sufficient in-service training and whether therapists are being encouraged to attend conferences and updating courses. Certainly some health authorities set aside few funds for this purpose.

There may be some potential for improving the effectiveness of therapists by decreasing the amount of time spent on administration and travelling between areas. Even a slight increase in the number of therapy staff (which would decrease the number of areas covered by individual therapists and reduce travelling time) or the appointment of a clerk to take over administrative duties, may have a benefit which is disproportionately greater than the cost.

Nevertheless most therapy time at present is spent with individual patients and very little in group activity. Even if more staff were available it seems unlikely that more patients would be treated, though the quality of treatment might improve. Therapists seem to be more concerned with increasing the amount of time on long-stay wards and in the community.

Although an increase in physiotherapy activity on long-stay wards is likely to result from an increase in staffing levels, it is not clear what this would achieve. If the aim is to improve the quality of life by increasing physical activity then the use of activities organisers and volunteers might be more appropriate. If, on the other hand, the goal is to improve the ability of long-stay patients to a level where they can be discharged to the community then increased physiotherapy would be productive. This would indicate, however, that rehabilitation at an earlier stage had not been adequate.

It does not seem that additional physiotherapy staff would result in more research into rehabilitation. This is understandable since few therapists have any experience of research techniques and rehabilitation is a particularly difficult field for research. It is essential, however, that present techniques are evaluated and new ones developed if physiotherapy is to gain greater respectability amongst fellow professionals. It is also essential for the advancement of the profession. In view of this it seems important that efforts are made to provide research posts for physiotherapists in specialist units.

9 Conclusions

Since geriatric medicine is a very broad specialty there is ample opportunity to develop an emphasis on special types of management. While all geriatricians must be expert at dealing with acute illness in old people, some will see this as their major interest while others will put greater emphasis on rehabilitation, long-stay care or community care. Inescapably, however, all of these aspects of geriatrics are the responsibility of each consultant and any of them is neglected only to the detriment of the service.

The development of an age-related policy will largely depend on the availability of resources and the attitude of other physicians. Some units, for instance, take responsibility for all acute admission of people over pensionable age (at present 60 for females and 65 for males) while others set limits such as 70, 75 or 85 years and over. It is questionable whether such clear cut-off points are desirable. To be 'general medical' on one day and 'geriatric' on the following day because of a birth date is irrational and bewildering to patients. In general this age-related policy applies only to emergency admissions and younger patients may be accepted on a secondary referral basis if the specialist skills of the geriatric unit are required or following a request for consultant advice by the general practitioner.

This interest in acute services for the elderly has encouraged the development of posts of general physician with an interest in (or responsibility for) the elderly. These posts will inevitably influence the style of practice of the geriatrician. The arguments for these posts are that they allow greater flexibility in the care of the elderly, the physician is able to enjoy a wider practice of his clinical skills, the relationship between geriatricians and general physicians is improved and rotation of junior medical staff between general medicine and geriatrics is facilitated. The contrary argument is that geriatric medicine is a full-time job if carried out properly, requiring an administrative and managerial role in organising the service and communicating with community services in addition to the wide range of clinical services to be provided. Involvement with acute emergencies in 20- and 30-year-olds as well may be more of a distraction than a benefit or, alternatively, the care of younger patients may take priority over the elderly when the pressure is on.

If, as is often stated, the acute aspects of geriatric medicine are no different from those in general medicine there would be no need for geriatricians to be concerned about their role in care of the acutely ill elderly person. Although some of this concern reflects their own need to be involved at the sharp end of medicine with all the fascination of investigation, diagnosis and treatment, there are certain features of illness in the elderly which warrant a specialist geriatric approach. The urgent presentation of disease may be a *de novo* acute episode, an acute exacerbation of a chronic illness (such as acute on chronic bronchitis), an acute presentation of a chronic disorder (such as falls) or an acute disorder presenting as an apparent chronic condition (such as acute chest infection presenting as confusion which is misdiagnosed as being of long standing). The traditional concept of multiple pathology—and the difficulty of deciding which symptom belongs to which disease and which condition requires treatment first, if at all—is well recognised. Multiple pathology is associated with the more insidious polypharmacy and this, along with changing pharmacokinetics and pharmacodynamics of advancing age, can cause great difficulty in diagnosis and management. There are also problems with different presentation in old age, such as the 'silent' myocardial infarction, apathetic thyrotoxicosis or apyrexial infections. On the other hand conditions such as confusion, falls, immobility or incontinence may be the presenting symptom of disease in almost any system in the body. Other difficulties arise in knowing whether a clinical feature is simply normal ageing or is pathological (for example, muscle wasting, absent ankle jerks or decreased vibration sense). Many conditions in the elderly present with non-specific symptoms such as tiredness and failure to thrive—usually diagnosed as 'old age' or 'senility'. Equally important is the fact that a successful outcome often depends as much on the effectiveness of discharge planning by the multidisciplinary team as on the medical treatment of the underlying condition. All of these complications increase the need for the geriatrician to be involved in the acute aspects of patient management.

Most geriatricians place great emphasis on looking after patients with complex problems associated with multiple pathology and social or psychological disadvantages. This has encouraged the development of rehabilitation services in most geriatric units. Since rehabilitation as a specialty has not really existed in the UK there has not been the same debate about who undertakes the rehabilitation of the elderly as there has been about the responsibility for acute care. This may change in the next decade as the attitude to district-based rehabilitation services changes.

Nevertheless, the management of disabling disorders of the elderly is central to geriatric practice. Special expertise in this area

Conclusions

has encouraged geriatricians in Britain to pioneer specialist stroke rehabilitation units. As we have shown, about 11 per cent of geriatric departments have a stroke unit. The advantages of these units include the concentration in a small area of specialist skills in the management of stroke and a nursing staff who understand the important principles of correct positioning to inhibit the dominant tonal pattern, protection of the shoulder and management of perceptual disorders and dysphasia. The evidence is[1] that patients are discharged from stroke rehabilitation units earlier, in a more independent state and having received less physiotherapy and occupational therapy time than those on a general ward. These units have been shown[2,3] to decrease both morbidity and mortality following strokes. Probably the person who benefits most[4,5] is the patient who has a severe (rather than profound) stroke. Stroke rehabilitation units are also more likely to be associated with volunteer support systems such as stroke clubs (social societies for the stroke victims and their families) or volunteer schemes for dysphasic patients[6] which provide volunteers who understand the problems of dysphasia and can work with dysphasic patients to help them, and their families, overcome the handicaps imposed by the communication problem[7].

The other specialist unit in which geriatricians have become involved, in cooperation with orthopaedic surgeons, is the geriatric-orthopaedic (GO) unit[8,9]. These have the advantage of providing a combination of medical, orthopaedic and rehabilitation components to the management of the elderly person with orthopaedic problems (especially fracture of the femoral neck). As can be seen from our studies about 20 per cent of geriatric units had some formal liaison with the orthopaedic department.

The long-stay sector of patient management is also undergoing changes in organisation. It is regrettable but true that long-stay care is to many geriatricians the least attractive part of their practice. On the other hand the long-stay ward has acted as a safety valve to control the build-up of pressure caused by 'blocked beds' on the acute and rehabilitation wards. For this reason most geriatricians have jealously guarded the right to control access to these valuable beds. This right is now under threat with the setting up of NHS nursing homes, albeit on an experimental basis, and the mushrooming of private rest and nursing homes. The danger is that lack of control of long-term care will have an adverse effect on the type of patient the geriatrician is likely to accept. He may welcome not having to accept the obvious long-stay patient from other specialists or from the community but will also be reluctant to risk attempting to rehabilitate a patient who may not respond to a level where he can return home. This may further encourage the emphasis on the acute aspects of geriatric management. However, many geriatricians take pride in the development of high quality long-term care facilities—and see this as the bedrock of their service.

Geriatricians have developed a number of styles of practice to manage the problems of the elderly. The commonest style is to combine acute and rehabilitation elements in one group of wards and long-stay patients in a separate group of wards. This style is most common in rural areas where there are several hospitals to be covered, probably because it is difficult to provide acute and rehabilitation services effectively in a number of small hospitals. There is also an advantage in providing long-stay care in small hospitals near to the patient's own home town. There may also be some advantage in combining the acute and rehabilitation elements of care since, as we have shown earlier, even units with wards designated specifically for rehabilitation admit a significant proportion of acute medical cases directly.

The main debate is between the combined (ARL) and the separated (A/R/L) units. In the ARL or 'mixed flow' style the acute, rehabilitation and long-stay elements of patient care are managed on every ward, whereas in the A/R/L or 'progressive care' style separate wards are designated for each element.

The advocates of the ARL style argue that it offers greater flexibility of beds so that the patient with the greatest need at the time gains admission to the bed. This should provide a more rapid turnover of patients and improve the discharge rate whereas those units with the A/R/L style are likely to have a waiting list for one type of ward while there are empty beds on another. The evidence from our studies does not support the argument that the A/R/L style is inefficient since, overall, units with this style had the highest turnover. This may be because in practice they admitted acutely ill patients to the rehabilitation wards when a bed was not available on the acute wards. There is some evidence for this from our studies.

Another advantage put forward for the ARL style is that it is more attractive to nurses since it 'dilutes the difficult patients' and therefore makes it easier to recruit staff to the long-stay elements of care. Others would argue that this is a negative approach and that it would be more appropriate to provide better care for the 'difficult' patient which in turn would attract nurses. One further suggested advantage of the ARL style is that patients who are slow to respond are encouraged by seeing others with similar conditions improve and therefore are stimulated to try harder. The opponents argue that the opposite is just as likely to apply—the patient becomes depressed at others progressing more quickly and therefore gives up trying. Both of these views are, of course, applicable whatever the style of the unit.

The advocates of the A/R/L style argue that each of these elements of care is fundamentally different, requiring specialist nurses in specialist environments with specialist equipment. The acute ward needs nurses who are trained in the management of acute illness, capable of understanding the high technology approach associated with general medical wards. They need the skills of monitoring acutely ill patients and coping with the various types of infusions, ECG monitoring and procedures such as pleural effusion aspirations, biopsies and sigmoidoscopy. Although many of these procedures can be carried out on any ward, having nurses conversant with the equipment and having the equipment easily available has its advantages.

Nurses on the rehabilitation ward need an educational (and educated) approach to patient management and require a different range of equipment (various types of walking aids, pneumatic intermittent compression machines, ultrasound and so on). The emphasis of the ward is on activities of daily living rather than medical-nursing models of practice.

The advocates of the A/R/L style argue that separate long-stay wards have the advantage of providing a more homely environment where there can be more social activity as well as more privacy: where the activities are recreational and relatives and volunteers can play an important part in improving the quality of life. The furniture is likely to be different with more soft furnishing, ornaments and pictures, and pets may be kept. The opponents of the style would argue that this can, and does, happen in some mixed flow wards whereas there are many long-stay wards which are totally depressing, with low levels of staff and patients either confined to bed or sitting beside the bed in night clothes for the entire day with no activity. Sadly we did see some such cases on our visits. We were also very impressed by the type of activity we found in some wards of all types. There are obviously good and bad units whatever the style.

One further argument put forward for the A/R/L style is that it allows greater efficiency in the use of scarce resources by concentrating these in small areas. The use of remedial services is one example of this. Certainly evidence from our studies suggests that, even using the guidelines derived from studies 3 and 4, there is a shortage of about 390 trained physiotherapists and about 590 trained occupational therapists for geriatric units in the UK, mostly in England. The evidence from studies 3 and 4 was that some therapists spent an unnecessary amount of time travelling between wards. No doubt some of this was due to the low level of staffing, a problem which may be relieved by having fewer wards to which the therapists have to travel.

The shortage of therapists is of major concern and with the numbers required will not be overcome in the foreseeable future. There is little scope for transfer of staff from other areas. The obvious solution would be to train more therapists but this is unlikely in the present economic climate. One of the problems is that while clinicians recognise that physiotherapy and occupational therapy are generally effective, there is almost no research evidence to support this view, largely because the research has not been done. As shown in our studies, therapists do not seem to be particularly interested in engaging in it, partly because of lack of training in rehabilitation research and the obvious attraction of so much direct patient contact. It is probably also due to the complexity of rehabilitation research. It does not easily lend itself either to the clinical trial format (since there is difficulty in using a double blind trial structure when the treatment involves a person) or to a crossover design in an educational model of treatment. The need for active cooperation from the patient, his family and others and difficulties in developing suitable measurements are other problems. Nevertheless, unless there is good research evidence for the effectiveness of rehabilitation techniques it is difficult to persuade health authorities to fund this expansion.

Other approaches are obviously required to ensure satisfactory rehabilitation management of patients. One suggestion is to encourage those therapists who are no longer working to return to clinical practice. The therapy professions have a high drop-out rate largely because they are dominated by females who leave to raise a family. An active campaign is needed to encourage these trained staff to return after their families have grown up and to provide reorientation courses for them. More males might also be encouraged to enter the therapy professions.

Finally, their efficiency could be maximised by concentrating their efforts where they can be shown to be most effective while training other professional groups to become involved in other areas of rehabilitation. Nurses are an obvious group to be trained in rehabilitation techniques: they are the only professionals who are responsible for 24-hour patient contact. Rehabilitation is a process of assisting the patient to learn to cope with daily activities and therefore needs to take place throughout the whole day. It is confusing to the patient to be taught one technique by the physiotherapist, another by the occupational therapist and yet another by the nurses. This is where interdisciplinary team work is

Conclusions

so effective. One of the common comments expressed on the questionnaires returned by physiotherapists and occupational therapists was that some nurses complicated the recovery process through lack of knowledge and an unduly 'caring' role. This highlights the need for special training at both the pre- and post-basic level for nurses, possibly with a special diploma in rehabilitation nursing. We would hope that in wards with a high rehabilitation input the charge nurse at least would have this certificate. These nurses would supervise patients' basic mobilisation and daily activities, thereby allowing the therapists to concentrate on the more complex and specialised techniques. All staff could then use their special skills to better effect. Training nurses in rehabilitation has special implications for community nurses now that community management of disabled people is the byword.

Therapists do have special skills and expertise both in physical techniques and in the use of equipment. The management of stroke is one obvious example. Nearly all the departments used one or more of the specialised neurophysiological approaches to stroke management—especially the Bobath concept. It was, however, obvious that therapists modified the techniques according to their own and the patients' needs. It is also obvious that there is a wide range in the approaches to rehabilitation of the elderly. This can be seen in the variable use of slings to prevent and treat the painful shoulder; calipers; pneumatic intermittent compression and the various types of walking aid in stroke rehabilitation. Similarly there is a wide variation in the involvement of the physiotherapist in the treatment of pressure sores. Such variation suggests a lack of information on the appropriateness of individual techniques and once again emphasises the need for more research into rehabilitation carried out in specialised centres.

Therapists felt that if more staff were available it was unlikely that more patients would be treated. This probably implies that most patients on geriatric wards who require rehabilitation receive at least some. More therapists would allow patients to receive treatment earlier and at a higher level.

It is interesting that both physiotherapists and occupational therapists indicated that if they had more staff they would increase their work on long-stay wards. The occupational therapists obviously saw their role in diversional activities and reality orientation as important though it is not too clear what the physiotherapists felt was their role. Presumably an exercise programme may help to keep patients healthier though whether this requires the skills of highly trained physiotherapists is debatable. Much of it could be carried out effectively by activities organisers who would develop expertise in the special needs of long-stay patients and use the services of unpaid volunteers. Indeed those units which we felt showed the most initiative in long-stay care had at least one member of staff (neither nurse nor therapist) whose role was to organise long-stay activities with the support of volunteers. One of the present difficulties in the UK is finding a suitable grade with a career structure for such appointments. Until this is accomplished an unnecessary barrier is being put in the way of departments wishing to appoint an activities organiser. Whatever the future aims of therapists it seems unlikely that there will be sufficient staff to deal with the needs of geriatric units.

Therapists are not the only resource which is underprovided. There can be no excuse for the very wide variations found for most other levels of provision as shown in these studies. For instance, 19 per cent of units in Engand had fewer than six beds per 1000 population 65 years and over while 23 per cent had more than 10.5 beds for an equivalent population; consultants in 28 per cent of units were responsible for fewer than 100 beds each whereas those in a further 24 per cent were responsible for over 160 beds each; there were 0.08 trained physiotherapists per 1000 population 65 years and over in one regional health authority and twice as many in another; and there is as much as a three- to fourfold difference between the number of beds per nurse in the top 20 per cent and those in the bottom 20 per cent of units. These differences are described only for England but there are similar variations in Wales, Scotland and Northern Ireland.

The situation is complicated further in that the four countries have developed their services based on different norms for resources. In England and Wales the 'norm' for the number of beds per 1000 population 65 years and over for many years has been 10 whereas in Scotland it is 15. Although there are problems in having set norms for the various resources there is a need for a planning base. It is essential that some guidelines are provided so that those departments with the lowest level of resources can be recognised and supported.

If, for instance, we look at the number of beds per 1000 population 65 years and over the evidence from our studies suggests that the discharge rate increases up to about 10 beds, then begins to decrease. Since most of the units with more than 10 beds per 1000 population were in those areas with greater responsibility for long-stay care (especially Scotland and Northern Ireland), it is understandable that the discharge rate should decline with increasing number of beds. More importantly, where there is low provision of beds there is also a low turnover. This again is understandable since

Conclusions

there will always be a core of patients who will require long-stay hospital care. The smaller the number of beds the greater proportion of those beds will be occupied by this group of patients. The findings from this study suggest that the optimal discharge rate occurs within the rate of 8.3 beds per 1000 population 65 years and over. This level should be universally provided unless there are very good local reasons for not doing so.

Tied in with the number of beds per population is the number of consultants per population and the number of beds per consultant. There are still a number of districts which have only one consultant for their geriatric service. In general these single-handed consultants are responsible for the largest number of beds per consultant, and have a low provision of other resources such as beds and physiotherapists per population. Not surprisingly they also have the lowest discharge rate per bed and per population. It would therefore seem important that a high priority be placed on ensuring that there are at least two consultant geriatricians in each district.

It would also seem important to examine the number of geriatricians related to the size of their client group. There was a wide range of provision varying from fewer than 0.04 to more than 0.11 consultants per population 65 years and over. In general the lower the number of consultants per population the poorer the turnover of patients. The optimal level of around 0.08 consultants per population would seem to be a reasonable minimum. This would reduce the number of beds for which some consultants are responsible. The general trend for turnover to decrease with increasing number of beds per consultant indicates that a consultant should not be responsible for more than 140 beds.

We have discussed these figures in terms of the population 65 years and over but it is essential that planning now be based on the population 75 years and over since this is the predominant age group in geriatric units (79 per cent of geriatric beds—Table 1). Taking the present bed occupancy by the different age and sex groups, and using demographic trends, it can be calculated that 14 per cent more beds will be needed in the next 15 years to provide a service equivalent to the present. This of course assumes no change in other provisions such as increased community care or private rest homes. The managerial expectations are that it will be possible to cut down the number of long-stay patients thereby increasing turnover through those beds. However, the greatest increase in bed requirements will be for long-stay beds (16–17 per cent for females) over the next 15 to 20 years. Since, overall, about 55 per cent of geriatric beds are used for long-stay care, a vast amount of increased services for the heavily physically and mentally elderly disabled outside hospital will be required. A reduction in the number of long-stay beds is therefore highly unlikely. The cost of caring for the heavily disabled in the community is as expensive as hospital care and carries a greater risk of poorer quality of care. There is also little evidence that the private sector is willing to cope with the type of patient who requires long-stay care. While transfer to private care decreases the cost to the local health authority, it is still costly to the country as a whole, especially since much of the funding is provided by public funds (£190 million in 1984).

All of this points to the need to plan on an age-related basis, taking into account local demographic trends and other resources. It seems appropriate to consider the number of beds and consultants in relationship to the size of the elderly population. For nurses the number of beds per nurse on duty is probably more important. As indicated earlier, there are wide variations in nurse staffing across the country. Staffing varies between districts, throughout the day, for different types of ward (acute wards having more nurses than those which are predominantly long-stay) and for the proportion of learners (more on acute wards than long-stay wards). Such a wide variation in nurse provision (amounting to more than 100 per cent difference between different districts) can have no rational basis. It probably reflects the varying availability of nurses for recruitment as well as the lack of a critical review of the work performed by nurses on geriatric wards. Our figures suggest that a staff ratio of 4.8 beds per nurse during the morning and afternoon, 6.9 at 7pm and 10 beds per nurse at night is the minimum requirement. These levels have still to be achieved in half the departments in the country.

Modern nursing philosophy with its patient-orientated approach (as opposed to task-orientated) is improving the quality of care and should be encouraged.

The predominant use of acute geriatric wards for the geriatric component of nurse training should be supplemented by work on rehabilitation and long-stay wards in order to provide student nurses with experience in these fundamental aspects of care of the elderly.

Perhaps the most striking overall finding to arise from these studies is the enormous inequality in the provision of resources between one health district and another. This applies to the supply of beds, as well as the numbers of medical, nursing and therapy staff. Such inequalities cannot be overcome without clear guidelines on the level of resources necessary to provide a geriatric service. One effect of reallocation within the health service has been to focus attention on those districts which are losing resources while overlooking districts which are underprovided. At the same time the movement of money between different districts will not of itself

Conclusions

ensure that it eventually finds its way to those areas in care of the elderly where need is greatest. Within nursing, for instance, additional resources may not reach the long-stay wards where they are so badly needed but become lost in district budgets, possibly moving to bolster acute services. Unless a checklist of guidelines is available it is hard to see how any rational planning can follow and it is likely that the most deprived areas of geriatrics will remain so. For this reason we believe that planning guidelines must be set on a national basis and that particular deficiencies in one area (for example psychogeriatrics) should be compensated for in another until they are corrected. Above average resources for geriatric medicine would thus be required in districts where the provision of residential homes or a psychogeriatric service is scanty. We also believe that there are limits to community care of isolated and disabled aged people. Where an effective geriatric service provides full facilities for medical assessment and rehabilitation with a high level of community liaison, careful screening of all long-stay patients will ensure that only those truly in need remain in hospital.

Our findings suggest that the following resource levels are minimal, assuming that other (non-geriatric) resources are adequate:

beds 22 per 1000 population aged 75 and over

consultant geriatricians 0.21 per 1000 population aged 75 and over and at least two geriatricians to each district

nurses a maximum of 4.8 beds per nurse in the morning and afternoon, 6.9 in the evening and 10 at night

trained occupational therapists 0.45 per 1000 population aged 75 and over

trained physiotherapists 0.47 per 1000 population aged 75 and over.

Finally, we have shown that a good deal of teaching is carried out in many geriatric departments. This includes medical students in the teaching hospitals, student nurses in most hospitals and students in the paramedical service, social services and others in many places. We have also indicated the need for considerable research on rehabilitation techniques and for the development of recreational activities for long-stay patients. With the present increasing move to the private sector, NHS geriatric departments may even see themselves providing these facilities for nursing homes on an agency basis. All of these activities require special centres devoted to research and training. Although this function naturally falls to academic geriatric units, past developments in geriatrics have taken place in notable centres remote from the teaching hospitals. We hope the pioneering endeavours of these centres will continue.

References

CHAPTER 1

1 Clarke M, Hughes A O, Dodd K J *et al*. The elderly in residential care: patterns of disability. Health Trends, 1979, 11: 17–20.
2 Dodd K, Clarke M and Palmer R L. Misplacement of the elderly in hospitals and residential homes: a survey and follow-up. Health Trends, 1980, 12: 74–6.
3 Grundy E and Arie T. Falling rate of provision of residential care for the elderly. British Medical Journal, 1982, 284:799–802.
4 Department of Health and Social Security. Statistics and Research Division. Meals services 1979 and 1981. A/F79/2 and A/F81/2. London, DHSS, 1979 and 1981.
5 Department of Health and Social Security. Statistics and Research Division. Staff of local authority social service departments 1979 and 1981. S/F79/1 and S/F81/1. London, DHSS, 1979 and 1981.

CHAPTER 2

1 Department of Health and Social Security. Health and personal social service statistics for England 1981. London, HMSO, 1982.
2 Sherman J. Gerrymandering geriatric beds. Health and Social Service Journal, 14 February 1985: 181.
3 Questions in the Commons. British Medical Journal, 1984, 288:576.
4 Office of Population Censuses and Surveys. Population projections 1981–2021. London, HMSO, 1984.
5 British Medical Association. Board of Science and Education. Report of the working party on services for the elderly. (Chairman: Sir Ferguson Anderson). London, BMA, 1976.
6 British Geriatrics Society. Memorandum on provision of geriatric services. BGS/3.82a. London, BGS, 1982.
7 Department of Health and Social Security. Report of a study on the respective roles of the general, acute and geriatric sectors in care of the elderly hospital patient. London, DHSS, 1981.

CHAPTER 3

1 Scottish Home and Health Department. Scottish Health Services Council. Medical rehabilitation: the pattern for the future. Edinburgh, HMSO, 1972.

References

2 Hyams D E. Psychological factors in rehabilitation of the elderly. Gerontologia Clinica, 1969, 11:129–136.
3 Office of Health Economics. Compendium of health statistics, 5th edition. London, OHE, 1984.
4 Brocklehurst J C, Andrews K, Richards B and Laycock P J. How much physical therapy for patients with stroke? British Medical Journal, 1978, 1:1307–1310.

CHAPTER 5

1 O'Brien T C, Joshi D M and Warren E W. No apology for geriatrics. British Medical Journal, 1973, 4:277–280.
2 Bagnall W E, Datta S R, Knox J and Horrocks P. Geriatric medicine in Hull: a comprehensive service. British Medical Journal, 1977, 2:102–104.

CHAPTER 6

1 Wells T. Problems in geriatric nursing care. Edinburgh, Churchill Livingstone, 1980.
2 Royal College of Nursing of the United Kingdom. Manpower availability: 7,8,15. London, RCN, 1981.
3 Miller A. A study of the dependency of elderly patients in wards using different methods of nursing care. Age and Ageing, 1985, 14: 132–38.
4 McFarlane of Llandaff Baroness and Castledine G. A guide to the practice of nursing using the nursing process. London, C V Mosby, 1982.
5 Magid S and Rhys Hearn C. Characteristics of geriatric patients as related to nursing needs. International Journal of Nursing Studies, 1981, 18; 97–106.
6 Godlove C, Dunn G and Wright H. Caring for old people in New York and London: the nurses' aide interviews. Journal of the Royal Society of Medicine, 1980, 73: 713–723.
7 Scottish Home and Health Department. Nursing workload per patient as a basis for staffing. Edinburgh, Scottish Home and Health Department, Scottish Health Service Studies 9, 1969.
8 Hill S N and Milnes J P. Nurses' education [letter]. British Medical Journal, 1985, 291: 545.

CHAPTER 7

1 British Medical Association. Board of Science and Education. Report of the working party on services for the elderly. (Chairman: Sir Ferguson Anderson). London, BMA, 1976.
2 British Geriatrics Society. Report on rehabilitation services. London, BGS, 1974.

3 College of Occupational Therapists. Recommended minimum standards for occupational therapy staff:patient ratios. London, College of Occupational Therapists, 1980.

CHAPTER 8

1 British Medical Association. Board of Science and Education. Report of the working party on services for the elderly. (Chairman: Sir Ferguson Anderson). London, BMA, 1976.
2 Wessex Regional Hospital Board. Report of working party on care of the elderly. Winchester, Wessex Regional Health Board, 1972.
3 British Geriatrics Society. Report on rehabilitation services. London, BGS, 1974.
4 Smith D S et al. Remedial therapy after stroke: a randomized controlled trial. British Medical Journal, 1981, 282: 517–520.

CHAPTER 9

1 Garraway W M, Akhtar A J, Prescott R J and Hockey L. Management of acute stroke in the elderly: preliminary results of a controlled trial. British Medical Journal, 1980, 280: 1040–43.
2 Drake W E, Hamilton M J, Carlson M and Blumenkrantz J. Acute stroke management and outcome: the value of a neurovascular care unit. Stroke, 1973, 4: 933–45.
3 Cooper S W, Olivet J A and Woolsey F M. Establishment and operation of combined intensive care units. New York State Journal of Medicine, 1972, 72: 2215–20.
4 Blower P and Ali S. A stroke unit in a district general hospital: the Greenwich experience. British Medical Journal, 1979, 2: 644–46.
5 McCann R C and Cuthbertson R A. Comparison of two systems for stroke rehabilitation in a general hospital. Journal of American Geriatrics Society, 1976, 24: 211–16.
6 Griffith V E and Miller C L. Volunteer stroke scheme for dysphasic patients with stroke. British Medical Journal, 1980, 281: 1605–7.
7 Lesser R and Watt M. Untrained community help in the rehabilitation of stroke sufferers with language disorders. British Medical Journal, 1978, 2: 1045–48.
8 Clarke A N G and Wainwright D. Management of fracture of the femur in the elderly female: a joint approach of orthopaedic surgery and geriatric medicine. Gerontologia Clinica, 1966, 8: 321–6.
9 Devas M B. Geriatric orthopaedics. Annals of Royal College of Surgeons of England, 1976, 58: 15–21.

Index

Activities of daily living
  aim of rehabilitation 35
  dependency on nursing staff 70–1
  role of occupational therapists 73, 82
  supply of aids 83–4, 85
  use of model kitchens/flats 73
Age of patients
  demographic factors 111–12
  on long-stay wards 45–6
  on rehabilitation wards 37–8
  related to admissions 103
  related to length of stay 20
Amputees
  admission to rehabilitation wards 39, 55
  length of stay on long-stay wards 46
  mobility aids 96
  rehabilitation, role of physiotherapists 86
Arthritis
  admission to rehabilitation wards 38, 39
  length of stay on long-stay wards 46
  rehabilitation, role of physiotherapists 86
Artificial limb and appliance centres (ALAC) 100
Assessment of needs 15, 16, 19
  before admission to long-stay wards 44, 47
  wheelchairs 100

Balance problems, admission to rehabilitation wards 38, 39

Beds 16
  DHSS norm 30
  future requirements 34
  long-stay 22
    related to discharges 23
  number per consultant geriatrician 24, 110, 111
  number per nurse 63, 110
    by type of geographical area 65, 67
    related to time of day 62, 112
    related to type of ward 62–3, 64–5
  occupancy rate 30
  provision
    by region 13, 21
    in regional ten-year plans 30
    related to community factors 31
    related to occupational therapy staff levels 79–80
  reduction in number 16, 30
  related to discharges 29, 31
  related to population 110–11
  relationship to discharges 29
  variations between countries 30–1, 110–11
  various types of unit 56–7
  suggested norms 33, 113
British Geriatrics Society recommendations
  consultant geriatrician numbers 32
  occupational therapy staffing levels 75–6
  physiotherapy staffing levels 86, 89, 101

117

British Medical Association
  recommendations
  consultant geriatrician
    numbers 32
  occupational therapy staffing
    levels 75–6
  physiotherapy staff levels 86,
    88, 101

Carcinomas
  admission to rehabilitation
    wards 39
  length of stay on long-stay
    wards 46
Community
  admissions to long-stay wards
    from 45
  liaison with 13, 31
    factor in planning 14
  role in rehabilitation 38
Confused patients, admission to
  rehabilitation wards 38, 39
Consultant geriatricians
  attitudes to rehabilitation 35
  first appointments made 15
  frequency of rounds in long-
    stay wards 48, 49, 52
  initial workload 15
  liaison with general physicians
    103
  management of patients in
    long-term care 44
  numbers 15, 19
    DHSS target 32
    future requirements 33–4
    norms 32
    per department 25
    related to available
      resources 25–6
    related to beds 24, 110, 111
      in various types of unit
        56–7
    related to discharge rate
      24–5, 33
    related to number of
      therapists 26, 27, 33
    related to population 23, 32
      in various types of unit
        56–7
    shortfall 33–4
    single-handed 33
    suggested norms 33, 113
  questionnaires 17
  responsibilities 19
  supervision of long-stay wards
    47–8

Day centres, seldom used for
  rehabilitation follow-up 41
Day hospitals 13, 16
  establishment 16
  factors influencing discharges
    30
  occupational therapy
    departments 74
  rehabilitation follow-up 41, 42
Deaths
  in long-stay wards 45
  in rehabilitation wards 39, 41
Demographic factors
  changes in upper age groups
    31
  community care provision 14
  in planning 111–12
  influence on bed provision 31
  influence on bed-days in
    rehabilitation wards 37–8
  influencing planning of
    rehabilitation units 43
  projected growth in over-75s
    34
Dependency, of geriatric
  patients on nursing staff 70–
  1
Depressed patients, admission
  to rehabilitation wards 39
Discharges
  as measure of efficiency 32

Index

from long-stay wards 45, 51
from rehabilitation wards 39
influence of short-term
  admissions 32
optimal rate 21–2
prior assessment home visits
  82
questionnaires 17
related to bed numbers 29, 31
  and beds per population 29
  in long-stay wards 23
related to consultant
  manpower 24–5, 33
  single-handed geriatricians
    33
related to type of ward 55–6,
  58
variations in countries of UK
  27–8

Falls, by patients on long-stay
  wards 47
Femurs, fractured
  admission to rehabilitation
    wards 38, 39, 55
  length of stay on long-stay
    wards 46
  rehabilitation 42
  role of physiotherapists 86

General practitioners
  involvement in long-stay
    wards 48
  involvement with prototype
    NHS nursing homes 48
  rehabilitation follow-up 41
Geriatric medicine
  acute illnesses 103–4
  appointment of general
    physicians 103
  contribution of occupational
    therapists 73
  diagnostic problems 104
  early days of NHS 15

elements 53
expansion 13
historical background 14–16
importance of rehabilitation
  35
range of services involved 13
regional variations 13, 19
role of consultant geriatricians
  19
specialist service development
  59
studies undertaken 16–18
variations in organisation 59–
  60
Geriatric units
  acute 13
  combined with
    rehabilitation and long-
    stay (ARL) 53–4, 60,
    106–7
  combined with
    rehabilitation (AR/L)
    53–4, 60
  occupational therapists
    78–9
  requirements 60
  with separate rehabilitation
    and long-stay (A/R/L)
    53–4, 60, 106–7
  efficiency assessment 58,
    60
  physiotherapists required
    91
  age-related admissions 103
  beds related to population 21
  differences in organisation
    53–4
  early days of NHS 15
  length of stay
    average 30
    related to type of ward 55–6
  long-stay 13
    access to beds 105
    activities organisers 110

119

(Geriatric units, long-stay, continued)
   admissions 44, 45
   age and sex distribution 45–6
   as separate wards 44, 53–4, 60, 106–7
   combined with acute and/or rehabilitation wards 44
   deaths 45
   discharges 45, 51
   frequency of consultant rounds 48, 49, 52
   length of stay 45, 46
      related to diagnosis 46
   measures of effectiveness 51
   medical involvement 46–8
   number of beds 31
   occupational therapy 109–10
   patients from rehabilitation wards 40, 41
   physiotherapy provision 86, 95, 102, 109–10
   quality of life 47, 48–51, 52
   questionnaires 17
   recreational activities 49–50, 51, 85
   requirements 60
   separate wards 53–4, 58, 60, 91, 106–7
   student nurse training 52, 71–2
   waiting lists 46
  number of consultant geriatricians 25
  physiotherapy equipment available 101–2
  questionnaires 17
  rehabilitation 13, 35
   acute medical cases 38, 39, 42
   age and sex distribution 37–8
   deaths 39, 41
   diagnoses of admissions 38–9
   discharges 39–40
      follow-up arrangements 41–2
   factors leading to decreasing need 38
   length of stay 37–8, 39–41
      related to placement on discharge 40
   liaison with orthopaedic wards 36, 42
   medical training 38, 42
   occupational therapists 79
   relief admissions 41
   requirements 60
   source of admissions 36
   student nurse training 72
   transfers from other wards 55
  sample visited 18
  sources of admissions to different ward types 54–5
  specialisation by hospitals 16
  staff levels, related to type of unit 58
  suggested norms 33
  training of medical and nursing staff 113
  transfers from other wards 55
  see also Beds; Consultant geriatricians; Nurses; Occupational therapists; Physiotherapists
Geriatricians *see* Consultant geriatricians
Geriatric-orthopaedic units 105

Heart disease, length of stay on long-stay wards 46
Home help service 14, 31
Home visits
  assessment prior to discharge 82

Index

by consultant geriatricians
in early days of NHS 15
by occupational therapists 81
see also Physiotherapists,
domiciliary
Homes *see* Residential homes
Hospital Centre, study of nurse
staffing levels 66, 68

Incontinence
admission to rehabilitation
wards 39
among patients on long-stay
wards 47

Long-term care 16, 19
changing patterns 105–6
historical background 44
number of beds 22, 31
questionnaires 17
reduced demand 16
see also Geriatric units, long-stay

Meals-on-wheels service 14, 31
Myocardial infarction,
admission to rehabilitation
wards 39

National Council of Nurses,
study of nurse staffing levels
66, 68
Neurological disorders,
rehabilitation 39, 42
Nurses
attitudes to recreational
activity involvement 51
dependency of geriatric
patients 70–1
factors influencing morale 68
in residential homes 14
included in study 18
involvement in long-term care
47

numbers
controversy 61
factors to be considered 66
related to number of beds
63, 110
at different times of day
62, 112
by type of geographical
area 65, 67
in different types of ward
62–3, 64–5, 71
study of staffing levels 61–6
suggested norms 113
primary nurse:patient ratio 69
ratio of trained to untrained/
learners 63, 65–6
relationship with patients 68
responsibilities of primary
nurses 68–9
students
numbers in different types
of ward 63, 66
on long-stay wards 52, 71–2
on rehabilitation wards 72
task-orientated and patient-
centred approaches 68, 112
training in rehabilitation 42,
77, 101, 108–9
Nursing homes
NHS prototypes 47–8, 105
see also Residential homes,
private

Occupational therapists
activities possible with more
staff 83, 84
aides 73–4
organising recreational
activities 49–50
related to number of
trained therapists 74–5
assessing need for wheelchairs
100

121

(Occupational therapists, continued)
  attitudes to recreational activity involvement 51
  combined with other therapy skills 78
  contribution to geriatric medicine 73
  development of departments 73
  home visits 81
  involvement in long-term care 47
  major function 73
  numbers 26, 27, 28, 74–5
    adequacy of staffing levels 75–8
    at present and required level 76
    related to elderly population 75–7
    related to number of consultant geriatricians 26, 27, 33
    related to type of unit 78–9
    related to workload 79–80
    shortfall 77
      possible remedies 84–5, 108–9
      suggested norms 113
    variations between countries of UK 77–8
  questionnaires 17
  research needs 108
  time spent on various activities 80–3
  training 73
Orthopaedic patients
  rehabilitation 36, 42, 59
    occupational therapists' involvement 74
  transfer to long-stay wards 45
  see also Geriatric-orthopaedic units
Outpatient departments, rehabilitation follow-up 41, 42

Parkinsonism
  admission to rehabilitation wards 39
  length of stay on long-stay wards 46
  rehabilitation, role of physiotherapists 86
Peripheral vascular disease, admission to rehabilitation wards 39
Physiotherapists
  activities possible with more staff 94–5
  aides 86, 88, 89–90
  assessing need for wheelchairs 100
  combined with other therapy skills 78
  domiciliary 13, 38, 86
  equipment available 95–7
  functions 86
  future training needs 90
  major activities 93, 102
  numbers 26, 27, 28, 110
    per bed 91
    perceptions of adequacy 87–9, 101
    related to number of consultant geriatricians 26, 27, 33
    related to type of area 91–2
    related to type of ward 91
    shortfall 89–90, 101
      possible remedies 108–9
    suggested norms 113
  preferred walking aids 96–7
  pressure sore therapy 97
  questionnaire 17, 86
  research needs 102, 108

workload 92–3
see also Stroke patients, rehabilitation
Pressure sores
  patients on long-stay wards 47
  therapy 97
Psychogeriatric services 16, 34, 59
  in long-stay wards 45
  occupational therapists' involvement 74

Quality of life, of patients on long-stay wards 47, 48–51, 52

Recreational activities 85
  in long-stay wards 49–50, 51
Regions
  bed provision 21
    related to consultant manpower 24
    ten-year plans 30
  distribution of consultant geriatricians 23
  distribution of therapists 27
  variations in geriatric medicine provision 13, 19, 30, 110–11
Rehabilitation 19
  changing approaches 104–5
  definition 35
  domiciliary 38
  early days of NHS 15
  follow-up arrangements 41–2
  multidisciplinary effort 35, 43
  questionnaires 17
  role of physiotherapists 86
  see also Geriatric units, rehabilitation; Stroke patients, rehabilitation
Relief admissions 13
  affecting discharge rate 32
  to long-stay wards 45
  to rehabilitation wards 41
Residential homes 16
  jointly funded with nursing care 14
  private 16, 34
    nursing homes 14, 31, 52, 105
    patients from rehabilitation wards 40
    problems caused for planning 14
    rest homes 14, 31, 105
  social service 31, 34
    care of dependent elderly 13–14
    factors in planning 14
    patients from rehabilitation wards 40
Resources
  facts sought from questionnaire 19
  in various types of geriatric unit 57
  need for national norms 34
  related to number of consultant geriatricians 25–6
  suggested norms 113
  variations in provision 110, 112–113
  see also Beds; Consultant geriatricians; Geriatric units; Nurses; Occupational therapists; Physiotherapists
Respiratory problems, admission to rehabilitation wards 39
Royal College of Nursing, study of nurse staffing levels 66, 68

Skin ulceration, admission to rehabilitation wards 39

Social services departments
   factors influencing discharges 29–30
   liaison with 13
   supply of aids to daily living 83–4, 85
   use of occupational therapists 73
   variations between countries of UK 13
   see also Residential homes, social service
Spinal pain, admission to rehabilitation wards 39
Stroke patients
   length of stay on long-stay wards 46
   rehabilitation 36, 38, 39, 42, 55, 59, 95
      developments 105
      length of treatment 41
      occupational therapists' involvement 74
      role of physiotherapists 86, 92–3
      training physiotherapists 102

Surgical patients
   admission to rehabilitation wards post-surgery 39
   transfer to long-stay wards 45

Therapists *see* Occupational therapists; Physiotherapists

Volunteer organisers, involvement in long-term care 47

Waiting lists
   disappearance 16
   early days of NHS 15
   for long-stay wards 46
Walking aids 96–7
Wards *see* Geriatric units
Warren, Marjorie 15
West Middlesex Hospital 15
Wheelchairs
   availability on long-stay wards 47
   provision 100
Workhouse infirmaries 15, 44

Younger-disabled units 59